MORINGA OLEIFERA:

Magic, Myth or Miracle

by

Dr. Howard W. Fisher

This book has been written as an educational tool. It is based upon a consensus of current facts contained in peer reviewed literature and the experience of the author. This book is not intended to be used for the purposes of diagnosing or treating diseases. The information provided herein should not replace the advice of your caregiver. Always consult your chosen informed health care practitioner for concerns of any symptoms or active disorders.

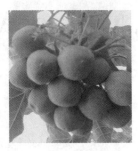

First Printed in Canada 2012
Britannia Printing
Toronto, ON, Canada
Copyright © 2012 by Dr. Howard Fisher

Fisher, Howard, Dr.
Moringa Oleifera: Magic, Myth or Miracle
Includes bibliographical references.
ISBN 978-0-9878218-0-5

This book is dedicated to the pursuit of knowledge in order to optimize health and well being.

Kannaeng doing (Thailand)

Murunkak-kai (Sri Lanka)

Malunggay (Philippines)

Horseradish tree (U.S.)

Chum Ngay (Vietnam)

Drumstick tree (U.K.)

Ben aile (France)

Sajna (India)

Mlonge (Kenya)

Nebeday (Senegal)

Benzolive (Haiti)

Dandalun (Burma)

Sitachini (Nepal)

Saijan (Pakistan)

Moringa

Table Of Contents

Table Of Contents

Table Of Contents

FOREWORD

"Invariably the simplest answer tends to be the correct one," as Ockham's Razor suggests. The simple answer, in this case, is the industrialized, processed, chemically refined, and genetically modified food and beverage chain, along with a tsunami of harmful drugs, is killing us. We are over fed, under nourished, and over drugged.

Dr. Fisher's treatise, that follows, is an incredibly well researched, succinct, and one hundred percent factual 'tour-de-force' on a botanical power-house called *Moringa Olifera*. The US National Institute of Health and Medicine, an official agency for the United States government, has affirmed Moringa can "arrest, reverse, and cure, over 300 different diseases and disorders". Big Pharma tried to develop this botanical into drug therapies, for decades, and failed.

There is an old Asian proverb that suggests "in every disaster there is opportunity"; efficacious Moringa is THE answer to a pandemic of nutrient depleted triggered conditions, and eliminates the need for useless, hyped, and dangerous drugs, that do not work, and/or harm.

Oh, by the way, Moringa radically improves wellness, with no intra-contradictions, at fractions of pennies on the dollar, with no adverse side effects. Benjamin Franklin, reminds each of us: "An ounce of prevention is worth a pound of cure"; Moringa is that ounce, literally.

I have been in the global food, beverage, confectionary, dairy, pharmaceutical, drug, bakery, cosmetic, flavor, as well as the functional and dietary supplementation formulation development business, for over three decades, and I have never come across a more nutrient dense botanical or raw material, in all my creation, conversion, or stabilization efforts, on six continents. *Moringa oleifera* is the real deal, and Dr. Fisher has put all the pertinent information, for your benefit, in this marvelous book!

In less than four decades, processed diets around the world have pushed the industrialized populations to one out of three individuals being insulin resistant, hyper or hypo glycemic, or type 1 or 2 diabetic. Seven out of ten in these industrialized food and beverage populations are literally obese or morbidly obese. The daily reports of inflammatory diseases, mental illness, cardio vascular diseases, and cancers, at abnormally high proportions, are a direct result of dumb-downed food and beverage chains.

Of the last 5,743 drugs approved at FDA, in America, in the last 25 years, the average number of adverse side effects, per drug, is at least 70.

We are, in great measure, what we eat, figuratively and literally. Said another way: It's The Food & Beverage Plus Drug Chains. Consume junk and take drugs; die early and in pain. Stupid! Provide for what the body requires, with nutrient dense Moringa; live long and well.

Moringa addresses, arrests, and reverses much that is broken, on so many levels, whether in deplete or void caloric intake, failed so-called health-care/sick-care systems, and/or so many reactive over-priced, evasive, and dangerous medical protocols, that do not work.

If we are to be judged by our talents bestowed and/or earned for the benefit of others, particularly the least among us, then Dr. Fisher has performed a great service for all humans on this planet in this seminal compendium, on this most rich botanical known to science and medicine.

To each of your best health and wellness!

Russell M. Bianchi
Managing Director & CEO
ADEPT SOLUTIONS, INC.
Soquel, California,
October 2011
www.russbianchi.com

PREFACE

As I watched the man, dressed in little more than a faded orange sarong, finish off his murky looking drink, he did a relatively strange thing. Strange, that is for, people from the western world. He dumped the last few milliliters into his hands and rubbed them around much like we would do with a hand sterilizer, that have become so popular since the outbreak of communicable diseases such as SARS, MRSA and flu epidemics. Next he rubbed his hands all over his face. He noticed me watching him intently and he looked at me and said "Sigru!" I did not make the connection at the time, but the man's skin, the lack of wrinkles and anticipated age lines, did not reflect his apparent age. His hair was as white as the snow covered Himalayas but I was at the complete other end of India in Kerala. I asked the guide what the man was drinking and he said something about a 'drumstick tree'. He called it 'Morunna,' a different name from the man drinking it and so now my curiosity was officially piqued.

When one examines the current state of world health and considers the rampant disease compounded by poor quality non-potable water and malnutrition, who would suspect that a tree that grows faster than most, might be the solution to the bulk of these problems? Many of us in this field have strongly suspected that the solution might come from the constantly reduced South American rainforest, but it appears that it is the 'drumstick tree' (*Moringa oleifera*), indigenous to the part of the world with the highest density of population, southern Asia and Africa.

More than two years ago when I first started to write this book, I knew that I was delving into an area in which the bulk of the general population needed more relevant information. Obesity in North America is running rampant. Just look around. You will start to realize that something is wrong and we need help. The cause is related to poor food choices or eating disorders, but eventually this leads to heart disease and diabetes.

I was well aware of the nutritional dangers that lurked in our midst and that was one of the reasons for dispensing this information. We are facing a crisis. I have been trying to fight against it adamantly for about the last two decades and hopefully I am holding my own. It is not an easy fight and quite frankly, we may need magic or a miracle simply because most people are looking for the easy way out. The truth of it is that to work at the preventive aspects of aging and the factors that may lead to disease, is in fact an effort.

The regimen involves proper diet (which for me, includes being a vegetarian) exercise, eating organic foods whenever possible, detoxifying daily, and consuming a copious quantity of supplements daily in an effort to counteract the negative effects of life. What if there were a path that just seemed to make this all a little easier? There has been a resurgence of fatal outcomes from "new and old infectious diseases."[1][2][3] As you will see when the state of world health is discussed in the first chapters, finding a potential miracle only made me more passionate about getting the word out.

We live in a toxic world where the easiest choices seem to lead to our current level of disease. Basically, it is just much easier to continue to produce lower quality foods that are easily accessible through mass marketing. Consequently the onus is on us to take responsibility for

---

[1] Barrett R, Kuzawa W, McDade T, Armelagos G J. "Emerging and Re-Emerging Infectious Diseases: The Third Epidemiological Transition". *Annu Rev Anthropol.* 1998; (27): p.247-71.
[2] Lewis K. "Multidrug resistance pumps in bacteria: variations on a theme". *Trends Biochem Sci.* 1994; 19(3): p.119-23.
[3] Swartz M N. "Hospital acquired infections: diseases with increasingly limited therapies". *Proc Natl Acad Sci USA.* 1994; 91(7): p.2420-27.

our own health. In a perfect world the choices would be easier: avoidance of all environmental toxins, while providing our bodies with all of the optimal nutritional necessities, however this task does not seem to be possible... or does it? This book will not deal with the multitude of economic or commercial implications of *Moringa oleifera*, but merely the documented health benefits that we may all derive by investigating this magical tree.

How many pharmaceutical medicines are based on plant life? How many tribal shamans knew about every plant in the rainforest and what they could be used for? Many of us assumed that tribal remedies were folklore based on myth. Hopefully some of those answers will be provided throughout the course of this book as we determine whether in fact *Moringa oleifera* is indeed magical, mythical or a miracle.

Dr. Howard W. Fisher

CHAPTER 1

THE OLD NEW SUPERFOOD

"Every human being is the author of his own health or disease"

Gautam Buddha

In recent years, an abundance of 'super foods', modern and ancient, have been newly discovered and many more rediscovered from the wisdom of the ages. Seemingly each new food to be promoted is the undisputed victor in a never ending competition to find the ultimate antioxidant, carrier of phytonutrients, immune booster and vitamin powerhouse. While some of these fruits and plants are truly remarkable, every single one of them pales vastly in comparison to *Moringa oleifera*. Often referred to as, "The Miracle Tree", *Moringa oleifera* is quite frankly nature's most perfect plant. In fact, it is the MVP of the plant world.

The leaves of this extraordinary tree contain seven times the vitamin C found in oranges, four times the calcium in milk, four times the vitamin A in carrots, three times the iron in spinach, three times the vitamin E of almonds, three times the potassium in bananas and two times the protein in milk.[4] That's right, you haven't misread and this abundance of vitamins and minerals is

---

[4] Ramachandran C, Peter K V, Gopalakrishnan P K. 1980, Drumstick (Moringa oleifera): A multipurpose Indian Vegetable. *Economic Botany*, 34 (3) p.276-283.

literally the tip of the iceberg. Chances are if you've investigated *Moringa oleifera* in the past you've read or heard this fact before and with good reason; because people are genuinely stunned and amazed when they first discover it. This buzz seems to be what many websites are talking about, but I am going to try to fit this information into the big puzzle of life.

Regular use of *Moringa oleifera* has been shown to: improve immune system function, digestive function, mental clarity, restful sleep, sexual desire and performance, healthier and younger looking skin, overall blood circulation, visual acuity and overall general physical well being. It also assists in maintaining healthy heart function, normalizing blood pressure, lowering and regulating cholesterol levels, alleviating diabetes and stabilizing normal blood sugar levels. It protects the liver from damage, shows immense anti-inflammatory qualities, inhibits the activation of lymphoma cells and helps the recovery of patients suffering from leukemia and dengue fever.[5] As well, Moringa has been shown to slow down the aging process, and assist the body with weight loss. In addition to all of this, *Moringa oleifera* provides all of the essential amino acids and vital vitamins. It contains several important minerals, is an incredibly powerful antioxidant, is high in fiber, fights cancerous cells, tumors, ulcers, epileptic seizures and cleanses and detoxifies the entire body.[6]

In short, Moringa has been called, the most powerful antioxidant on earth (with over 46 naturally occurring antioxidants found in the plant itself), the most effective natural medicine to combat chronic disease and

---

5

[6] Paliwal R, Sharma V, Pracheta V. A review on Horse Radiah Tree (Moringa oleifera): A Multipurpose Tree with High Economic and Commercial Importance. *Asian Journal of Biotechnology*. 2011;3(4):p.317-328.

also the most nutritional plant ever discovered. The above lists are, in actuality, a fraction of the incredible and factual benefits of a plant that has been shown to fight everything from the common cold to cancer and has been so aptly named, "The Miracle Tree," although it probably sounds like snake oil right now.

This incredible plant, which is currently gaining in popularity and use in the western world, has been in constant use for thousands of years in the Himalayan foothills, the surrounding areas in India and Pakistan, and can even be traced back through history to the ancient Greeks, Romans and Egyptians. In the past, traditional Ayurvedic Medicine has used Moringa in the treatment of over three hundred diseases. The list ranges from anxiety and skin infections to scurvy and venomous snake bites. While every single ancient use might not have been the most directed and scientifically proven, these healers saw results and knew what an incredible panacea they had on their hands.

Over time the nutritional value and importance of *Moringa oleifera* was noticed and has led to the transplantation and naturalization of this plant all across the world. It is currently being grown in, "India, Pakistan, Afghanistan, Bangladesh, Sri Lanka, Southeast Asia, West Asia, the Arabian peninsula, East and West Africa, Southern Florida, throughout the West Indies, and from Mexico to Peru, Paraguay and Brazil."[7] This hardy tree needs very little water and can thrive in less than ideal conditions, as long as the temperature is warm enough. In every region across the earth that Moringa has found purchase, the local communities have discovered its

---

[7] Paliwal R, Sharma V, Pracheta V. A review on Horse Radiah Tree (Moringa oleifera): A Multipurpose Tree with High Economic and Commercial Importance. *Asian Journal of Biotechnology.* 2011;3(4):p.317.

multitude of uses, and more often than not, the plant has become seamlessly imbedded in their daily cultural use.

Moringa oleifera is commonly referred to as the "Drumstick tree" due to the drumstick like shape of its seed bearing pods, "Horseradish tree" due to the spicy hot flavor of its roots, and also "Mother's best friend," in east Africa due to its multitude of useful purposes. Globally, Moringa has a unique name from every country it can be found in and in some countries, a new title for every region in which it can be found. Some examples of *Moringa oleifera* other names are: "La Mu" in Mandarin, "Malunggay" in Tagalog, "Sahjan" in Hindi, "Murungai Maram" in Tamil, "Sajiwan" in Nepali. This humble and hardy tree is known by at least two hundred different names in various regions across the globe and is used for an even greater number of modern purposes.

As if the sheer versatility and varied use of this plant weren't enough, virtually every part of the Moringa tree from the roots to the flowers can be eaten or used. As mentioned earlier, Moringa is often referred to as the 'drumstick' tree, due to the shape of the unripe green pods that are most often used as a food source. These vegetable-like 'drumstick' pods are cooked in a wide variety of ways and consumed on a daily basis in India and Sri Lanka. The 'drumsticks' are prepared in a similar fashion to green beans and have a flavor reminiscent of asparagus. The flowers of the Moringa tree are high in calcium and potassium and only edible after being cooked. They have a taste similar to mushrooms.

The seeds of the tree can be roasted or even eaten raw like peas or pressed into oil. Ben oil (called this due to its high behenic acid content) is a clear, odorless oil derived from the seeds of the Moringa plant. This oil is very similar in nutritional value to that of olive oil and can be used in cooking as well as directly applied to the skin. Ben oil is being noted for its high antioxidant and nutrient content and is finding a much greater use in hair conditioner and anti-aging skin products. There is also the future potential to use the Moringa seeds as a viable source for biodiesel. I will not be discussing these parameters in depth as the focus of this book will be on the nutritional health aspects. The remaining seed cake left after oil extraction is also used as an agricultural fertilizer. This seed cake can also be used to purify drinking water as the cake itself contains the active components to remove solid particles from contaminated water. During this process, the bacteria attaches itself to the particles being removed from the water, making the seed cake an effective bacterial removal system.

Historically the root of the tree was mashed and used as a condiment similar to horseradish. This practice is now discouraged as the roots have been found to be very high in the alkaloid spirochin. While fatal in very large doses, the same alkaloid has been shown to carry antibacterial qualities in smaller amounts.

The leaves of the tree are used in a number of ways ranging from salads, soups, curries, sauces and in some places even pickled. Most commonly the leaves are treated in a similar fashion to spinach and are especially popular in the Philippines, South India and Africa. These fresh leaves are often dried and saved for later use in teas, powders, and seasonings. The dried leaves, in powder form, can be stored for a number of months and remarkably suffer from little to no loss in nutritional value.

In the past it simply wasn't practical or even possible for people living outside of countries or regions that were home to the Moringa tree to eat the various fresh pods, seeds and leaves of the plant on a daily basis. Luckily, modern technology has made it incredibly easy to incorporate the vast benefits of this plant and its wide range of phytonutrients into our diet through the form of a *Moringa oleifera* supplement or tea.

Due to the ease of cultivation and local production, the Moringa tree has found a new role and purpose in saving people's lives from poverty and hunger in developing countries. Due to its incredible vitamin and nutrient qualities, Trees for life, Church World Service and Educational Concerns for Hunger Organization are promoting *Moringa oleifera* as "natural nutrition for the tropics." The dried and powdered leaves along with other Moringa supplements are currently being used to treat malnourished children, mothers and HIV/AIDS patients in third world nations.[8] The results have been staggering. By crushing up the leaves and adding them to a porridge like mixture on a daily basis, severely malnourished children have made significant weight gains with the leaves now added to their diets.

Studies have been done on nursing mothers who were not producing enough milk to effectively feed and cover all of the nutritional needs of themselves and their children. With the addition of six tablespoons of leaf powder into their daily diets, nursing mothers received complete coverage of their daily iron and calcium needs, and also have been shown to produce significantly more breast milk for their children. Among its many intrinsic nutritional values, studies have shown that with a daily intake of *Moringa oleifera*, the body's immune system is stimulated and significantly bolstered. With regards to this specific function, Moringa supplements are now being given to patients suffering from HIV/AIDS in Africa. You may have heard all of this before, and you suddenly realize that you are not in Africa, so what health issues could possibly lead us to want to include this obviously potent plant as part of our daily diet? Let's find out.

---

[8] Prazuck T, Tall F, Nacro B, Rochereau A, Traore A, Sanou T, Malkin J E, Apaire-Marchais V, Masson D, Dublanchet et al. HIV Infection and Severe Malnutrition: A Clinical and Epidemiological Study in Burkina Faso. *AIDS*. 1993;Jan:7(1):p.103-8

CHAPTER II

YOUR HEALTH CHALLENGES

"Extreme remedies are very appropriate for extreme diseases."

Hippocrates

I remember it very clearly although it happened a little more than two decades ago. I stepped into my waiting room as a seventy-five year old patient was just leaving and I motioned the young testosterone filled twenty-year old patient to enter. We sat in my office and his first words were classic. "I never want to be that old. I'm going to live hard and die young. I don't want to be like that."

It was to be one of my first lectures about how everyone is different and that both environments, internal and external would have a much greater impact on how a person ages. "Fifty is the new thirty," I said. "What if you didn't have to be like that at seventy-five?" "What if you could shift from a chronological clock to a physiological clock?"

He looked puzzled and could only utter a monosyllabic, "Wha?". It was obvious to any observer that this seventy-five year old who was riddled with osteoarthritis, a former smoker whose swollen legs displayed the onset of congestive heart disease was not the poster boy for anti-aging medicine. I asked, "What if you could control how you age and be active, healthy and in no pain at his age?"

"He was decrepit man! I just don't want to be that way!"

This innocent conversation, trying to change the outlook of a young man's views on aging, perhaps best outlines the task we all face if we choose to control our own physiological clock. It has been one of my objectives as an anti-aging physician to tackle this task from the preventive aspect. Many of my colleagues are involved in the aesthetic aspects of aging where a nip here or a tuck there alone or in combination with a platelet or botox injection can make you appear decades younger.

Others are involved with the remarkable bio-identical hormone replacement therapy where they monitor your hormone levels and supplement in an optimal level manner before waiting for an out-and-out deficiency to occur. I prefer to work with a lifestyle game plan that involves a modification of how we treat ourselves or how we age from the inside. A few years ago, I had the privilege of addressing my colleagues at a medical conference at the Royal Society of Medicine in London, England. While attending one of the lectures at the conference, Prof. Dr. Helena Baranova asked the one hundred and ten doctors in the lecture hall to speculate on the relationship between the environment and disease. Only one was foolish enough to raise their hand and that of course was me. Being relatively well-read and researched, I replied, "Seventy-five to ninety percent of disease is environmental."

Dr. Baranova replied, "That is a good answer, but not the right answer. Eighty-five to ninety six percent of disease is caused by environmental factors." This fact is one that should make everyone reading this book immediately feel that they have more control over their health and the rate at which they are aging. Being aware of your environmental challenges will allow you to affect the influence they have on your physiological clock. Short of being one of those four to fifteen percent of the population suffering from a genetic disorder, you can take control of your health.

Anti-aging medicine actually only became a discipline about twenty years ago, although it was almost three decades ago when this journey to approach health from a natural perspective started; everyone knew that the task would be arduous. We have all heard of or seen the movies *Supersize Me* and *Food Inc.* and realize the challenges that exist merely from a nutritional perspective alone. The 'near death' condition experienced by eating three meals a day at McDonalds caused the fast food giant to review their menu. "Food Inc." freaked out more than a few people with their discovery of the 'forty-five day from egg to supermarket' chickens.

TABLE I
CURRENT HEALTH STATUS IN AMERICA

DISEASE	INCIDENCE
OVERWEIGHT/OBESE	180,000,000
SEASONAL ALLERGIES	60,000,000
CARDIOVASCULAR DISEASE	40,000,000
ARTHRITIS	37,000,000
SINUS PROBLEMS	30,000,000
DIABETES	23,000,000
ASTHMA	20,000,000
CANCER	12,000,000
ALZHEIMER'S	6,1000,000
TOTAL	**398,100,000**
U.S. POPULATION	308,000,000

The covert nature of the industrial toxicity in combination with the capitalistic big business ideology, are challenges that must be overcome. As the level of additives in our environment increases, the goal of wellness becomes more difficult to obtain, and yet the bulk of the population is either trying to keep their head above the fiscal water line, or does not have a strategy to cope.

The status of health in the western world is under attack from a multitude of sources and as we can see from Table I, this is leading to an increased incidence of disease. With a population of 308,000,000, the statistics indicate that there are more than 398,000,000 incidents of disease scattered among them.[9] Not only are people living in western countries being effected by disease, they are dying from them too. According to the United States Centers for Disease Control and Prevention, Department of Statistics (2007), the top causes of death are:

Cardiovascular disease (616,067)
Cancer (562,875)
Stroke (135,952)
Chronic lower respiratory diseases (127,924)
Accidents (123,706)
Alzheimer's Disease (74,632)
Diabetes (71,382)
Influenza and Pneumonia (52,717)
Nephritis, Nephrotic Syndrome (46,448).[10]

Aside from accidents, the majority of these chronic diseases effect the quality of life, decrease life expectancy and cause premature death. These maladies create a huge economic impact throughout their etiologies, and many of them can be affected by dietary and supplementation

---

[9] Adams P F, Martinez M E, Vickerie J L. *Summary Health Statistics for the U.S. Population: National Health Interview Survey*, 2009. National Center for Health Statistics. Vital Health Stat 10(248). 2010.
[10] U.S. Department of Health and Human Service Centers for Disease Control and Prevention. National Center for Health Statistics. Deaths – Leading Causes 2009. http://www.cdc.gov/nchs/fastats/lcod.htm.

choices, especially if we realize that there is a large nutritional impact on immune system function.[11] [12] [13] [14] [15]

The concept of wellness is one that must be embraced from all aspects in order to achieve optimal health. Most people do not realize the number of microorganisms and toxic pollutants that fill all aspects of our environment, tax our immune systems and the subsequent cumulative effects on our health. Sadly, technological and industrial advances have led to more potent chemical toxins being released into our ecosystems. "A toxin is basically any substance that creates irritating and or harmful effects in the body, undermining our health or stressing our biochemical or organ functions."[16]

There is no denying that with the current state of affairs, toxins now accumulate in our bodies more rapidly than the four major pathways of detoxification (feces, urine, perspiration and exhalation) can evacuate them. Fortunately the media, exponentially enhanced by the internet, spurred on by the threat of global warming, is now shedding some

---

[11] Fairfield K M, Fletcher R H. Vitamins for chronic disease prevention in adults: scientific review. *JAMA*. 2002; 287(23):p3116-26.
[12] Selhub J, Jacques PF, Rosenberg IH et al. Serum total homocysteine concentrations in the third National Health and Nutrition Examination Survey (1991-1994); population reference ranges and contribution of vitamin status to high serum concentrations. *Ann Intern Med*. 1999; 131: p331-339.
[13] Chandra RK. Influence of multinutrient supplement on immune responses and infection-related illness in 50-65 year old individuals. *Nutr Res*. 2002;22;p5-11.
[14] Knekt P, Reunanen A, Jarvinen R, Seppanen R, et al Antioxidant vitamin intake and coronary mortality in a longitudinal study. *Am J Epidemiol*. 1994; 139:p180-189.
[15] Ness A R, Powles J W. Fruit and vegetables, and cardiovascular disease: a review. *Int J Epidemiol*. 1997; 26:p1-13.
[16] Haas, Elson M. Stayin`g Healthy With Nutrition: The Complete Guide to Diet and Nutritional Medicine. Berkeley, California. Celestial Arts. 1992. p906.

light on the current status of this soon-to-be overwhelming environmental toxicity.

When the toxic load becomes too much for these systems, physiological changes in the form of dysfunctional or inappropriate responses cause the body to function incorrectly from an immunological,[17] [18] neurological,[19] and hormonal[20] [21] perspective. The bulk of the population has already been adversely affected. Those of us who are a little older contain more of the recently banned toxic chemicals than younger people.[22]

Toxins may exert their effects rapidly, such as drugs or chemicals, or over a long- term basis such as the mesotheliomas from inhaled particulate matter by miners. Even long term exposure to organochlorine compounds (OCCs) have been closely associated with infertility and miscarriages.[23] The absolute reality is that if we exceed the physiological levels of toxic tolerance, systemic disorders will occur. A direct connection between environmental toxic chemicals and birth defects, cancer, reproductive

---

[17] Vojdani A, Ghoneum M, Brautbar N. "Immune alteration associated with exposure to toxic chemicals." Toxicol Ind Health. 1992; 8:p239-253.
[18] Selgrade M K, Coopr G S, Germolec D R, Heindel J J. "Linking Environmental agents to autoimmune disease." Environ Health Perspect. 1999; 107: pS5811-S811.
[19] Haschek W M, Rousseaux C G. Handbook of Toxicologic Pathology. San Diego. Academic Press. 1991.
[20] Anderson H A, Lilis R, Selikoff I J et al. "Unanticipated prevelance of symptoms among dairy farmers in Michigan and Wisconsin." Environ Health Perspect. 1978; 23: p217-226.
[21] Haschek W M, Rousseaux C G. Handbook of Toxicologic Pathology. San Diego. Academic Press. 1991.
[22] Neumann J, Winterton S, Foulds J, Smith R, Lu J. Toxic Nation: A Report on Pollution In Canadians. Environmental Defence. 2005;p.16.
[23] Leoni V, Fabiani L, Marinelli G, et al. "PCB and other organochlorine compounds in blood of women with or without miscarriage: a hypothesis of correlation." Ecotoxicol Environ Saf. 1989; 17.p1-11.

problems, respiratory disorders and neurological dysfunction has already been well established.[24]

Just so you understand the magnitude of the problem, we have reached the stage where xenobiotics, chemicals foreign to the biologic system,[25] are present in the adipose tissue (fat) of 100% of the population.[26] It's not like there is any shortage of potential toxicity with the constant presence of pesticides, food additives, heavy metals, pharmaceuticals, alcohol, tobacco, caffeine and recreational drugs readily available for absorption in our environment. The body tries to eliminate as many of these chemicals as possible, so when they are present in the blood, the body makes its best effort to excrete them in urine and feces. When there is an excess, the body stores these unwanted toxins in fat and generally the fat deposits remain farther away from the most important organs.

In 1976, the Environmental Protective Agency initiated a program, the National Human Adipose Tissue Survey (NHATS), which assayed tissue samples for the presence of toxins. Their findings have shown that every sample tested showed the presence of styrene, 1,4 dichlorobenzene (moth balls), xylene, ethylphenol and OCCD (dioxin). Furthermore, another nine chemicals were found in more than 90% of the population. These included toxins such as toluene, dioxins, DDE and carcinogens such as benzene, chlorobenzene, and ethylbenzene. (DDE is a breakdown product of DDT).[27] Toxicity mostly affects the

---

[24] Neumann J, Winterton S, Foulds J, Smith R, Lu J. Toxic Nation: A Report on Pollution In Canadians. Environmental Defence. 2005; p.4.
[25] Friel J P, ed. Dorland's Illustrated Medical Dictionary. Twenty-fifth Edition. W.B. Saunders. Philadelphia. 1974.
[26] Gunderson E L. FDA Total Diet Survey, April 1982-April 1986, Dietary intakes of pesticides, selected elements and other chemicals. Food and Drug Administration, Division of Contaminants Chemistry. Washington, DC 20204.
[27] Crinnion W J. "Environmental Medicine, Part 1: The Human Burden of Environmental Toxins and Their Common Health Effects." Altern Med Rev. 2000; 5(1):p52-63.

than three decades since DDT usage was banned, however the population is still showing chemical toxicity from this pesticide. Many other countries, whose products we import, still use these pesticides and of course the wind still blows.

Although trillions of reactions occur within the body with every instant, the human body is basically only trying to carry out the functions for survival and it does so with a hierarchy. Nutrition is at the top of the physiological triage list of the body for a number of reasons, but most importantly because if the ingested food were not digested, it would putrefy and create a septic situation that could end up as more than a potential problem for the body. When the nutrients are no longer provided (no intake=no digestion), the bodily functions will shut down due to lack of energy and entropy, and eventual death, would result.

The human body requires a significant amount of nutrition to supply all of the physiological needs and therefore the action of digestion and assimilation take both a great deal of time and energy. The digestion of a moderate size meal uses the equivalent energy expenditure to a twenty-five mile walk (it is no wonder as to why enzymes play such a formidable role in our health). Most of an individual's energy is expended during the digestion phase and this is why people who eat large, heavy meals often feel lethargic.

Your body must digest the food, absorb the nutrients and evacuate the waste. This is our daily elimination cycle,[29] the time when your body is literally trying to take out the garbage, properly known as detoxification. Bowel movements and bladder function are only a small part of the toxin removal necessary for a healthy existence. Sweat glands are constantly laboring in an attempt to reduce the

---

[29] Haas, Elson M. Staying Healthy With Nutrition: The Complete Guide to Diet and Nutritional Medicine. Berkeley, California. Celestial Arts. 1992. p906.

toxic load on our body; our lungs are continuously exhaling contaminant gases and the lymphatic system is constantly removing toxic wastes.   Toxicity mostly affects the immune, endocrine and neurological systems causing almost any disorder.

When the toxic load becomes too much for these systems, physiological changes in the form of inappropriate responses cause the body to function incorrectly from an immunological,[30] [31] neurological,[32] and hormonal[33] [34] perspective. Yet our bodies are phenomenal works of superb engineering. Regeneration is not only a function of arthropods such as crayfish and other crustaceans. If you surf the web you will find hundreds, if not thousands of cases of people who have lost a digit that has grown back completely, nail and all. Humans have the ability to regenerate and do so on a regular basis. The secret is a combination of our nutrition strengthening our organ systems and our bodies having enough energy to complete the task. The unfortunate reality is that very few of us ever achieve a significant enough state of detoxification to regenerate.   If the body has the energy after digestion/assimilation and detoxification, it will attempt to regenerate. Our environments (both internal and external) have us constantly under attack and from the current incidence of disease in our population. It is time to look for a solution.

---

[30] Vojdani A, Ghoneum M, Brautbar N. Immune alteration associated with exposure to toxic chemicals. Toxicol Ind Health. 1992; 8:p239-253.
[31] Selgrade M K, Coopr G S, Germolec D R, Heindel J J. Linking Environmental agents to autoimmune disease. Environ Health Perspect. 1999; 107: pS5811-S811.
[32] Haschek W M, Rousseaux C G. Handbook of Toxicologic Pathology. San Diego. Academic Press. 1991.
[33] Anderson H A, Lilis R, Selikoff I J et al. Unanticipated prevelance of symptoms among dairy farmers in Michigan and Wisconsin. Environ Health Perspect. 1978; 23: p217-226.
[34] Haschek W M, Rousseaux C G. Handbook of Toxicologic Pathology. San Diego. Academic Press. 1991.

CHAPTER 3

THE RELATIONSHIP BETWEEN NUTRITION, HEALTH & MORINGA

"The doctor of the future will no longer treat the human frame with drugs, but rather will cure and prevent disease with nutrition."

Thomas Alva Edison
Inventor, Scientist

Nutrition is a major factor affecting our immune system.[35] Poor nutrition may create an absolute deficiency in factors, or co-factors of physiological functions that may result in problems such as a calcium magnesium imbalance resulting in muscle spasms or decreased calcium leading to osteoporosis.[36]

It is quite common, with the processed acidic nature of North American diets, to create an acidic environment shutting down enzyme systems. This may lead to any number of problems as simple as indigestion or as serious as inflammatory processes in the digestive tract causing the villi to have impaired absorption (Irritable Bowel Syndrome, Enteritis). Prolonged incomplete or improper digestion leads to impacted feces blocking absorption and

---

[35] Chandra RK. Nutrition and the Immune System; an introduction. Am J Clin Nutr. 1997; 66:460S-463S.
[36] Dawson-Hughes B et al. Effect of calcium and vitamin supplementation on bone density in men and women 65 years of age and older. New Engl J Med. 1997; 337:p670-676.

potentially creating a malabsorption syndrome thus causing
liver toxicity because the body is trying to reabsorb what it
believes to be nutrients in your colon. According to Dr.
Charles B. Simone, nationally renowned Medical
Oncologist and Immunologist, "nutritional deficiencies
decrease a person's capacity to resist infection and its
consequences and decrease the capability of the immune
system."[37]

Choosing food wisely and eating a balanced diet,
while avoiding fried foods and refined sugar, rice, and
flour, will help. However the vast majority of the
population consumes less than sixty-six percent (66%) of
the recommended daily allowance for one or more
nutrients.[38] An American study concluded that only nine
percent (9%) of the population consumed the recommended
five servings of fruit and vegetables daily and fifty percent
(50%) had less than fifty percent (50%) of the RDA of
vitamins A, C, E, and other nutrients.[39] Remember that the
recommended daily allowance is the minimum quantity of
a nutrient necessary to prevent a deficiency syndrome.

There are all manner of supplements that can help
to prevent these situations from occurring. Consider
chlorophyll containing greens, antioxidants, enzymes,
omega 3 fatty acids (fish oil, flax seed, hemp seed) and
colon cleansers as a minimum to help supplement your diet.
Remember that the word supplement means to replace what
is missing and sadly since the great depression, our food
sources have been deficient in both vitamins and minerals.[40]

[37] Simone C. Cancer & Nutrition. Garden City Park, New York.
Avery Publishing Group. 1992; p46.
[38] Murphy SP et al. Demographic and economic factors associated
with dietary quality for adults in 1987-1988 Nationwide Food
Consumption Survey. J Am Diet Assn. 1992; 92:1352-1357.
[39] Challem, Jack. 10 Reasons to take supplements. Aloha, Ore. The
Nutrition Reporter. October/November 1996; p7-9.
[40] Beach Rex. Modern Miracle Men. Washington. United States
Government Printing Office Document No. 264. 1941.

Harvesting and shipping modes do not take nutrition into account and in combination with extensive processing, improper storage and soil deficiencies, it is almost impossible to get adequate nutrition from our current food supply.[41]   There is a great deal of evidence supporting supplementation and the consequent decreased risk of diseases.   According to the Council for Responsible Nutrition, "There is ample evidence to suggest that the public will benefit from the adoption of healthy dietary patterns and healthy lifestyle habits including the regular use of nutritional supplements."[42]

There are literally hundreds of peer reviewed papers examining the phytonutrients and bioactivity of *Moringa oleifera* and the relationship to health.   The body of science relating nutrition to health has also expanded to the extent that pharmaceutical intervention has taken a back seat for a number of disorders. As can be seen from the statistics about the incidence of disease in the previous chapter, we are not doing so well.

For centuries man has known that there are direct causal relationships between nutrition, disease and aging. Sailors setting out to discover the new world would suffer from scurvy caused by a deficiency of Vitamin C.   Other diseases, such as rickets (Vitamin D), beriberi (Thiamin, Vitamin B1), and pellagra (Niacin, Vitamin B3) are unquestionably caused by vitamin deficiencies.   Research has linked many chronic diseases to significantly reduced intake, impaired absorption or decreased endogenous production of vital nutrients that act physiologically in our bodies to maintain a non-disease state of homeostasis when present at optimal levels.

---

[41] Balch J, Balch P. Prescription for Nutritional Healing. New York. Avery Publishing Group. 2000; p14.
[42] Dickinson A, Ed. The Benefits of Nutritional Supplements. Washington. Council for Responsible Nutrition. 1998; p61.

"Inadequate intake of several vitamins has been linked to chronic diseases, including coronary heart disease, cancer and osteoporosis."[43] The goal of this chapter is to examine the morbidity associated with aging and chronic disease[44] to determine the potential benefits of nutritional intervention and illustrate how Moringa will affect the health equation.

In the beginning of the last century, medical investigative pioneers such as Dr. Alexis Carrel, Nobel Prize winner in Physiology or Medicine for his vascular suturing and transplant techniques, had been seeking the answers to questions about life, aging, and cellular longevity. In 1912, while at the Rockefeller Institute, Carrel proved the virtual immortality of the cell by growing a small piece of chicken cardiac tissue in a nutritive medium solution. The tissue was transferred to another fresh batch of nutrient medium every forty-eight hours for more than thirty-two years.[45] The cells expired only upon the failure of the lab technician to add proper nutrients and to detoxify the fluid that surrounded it by changing the containers.[46] Based on these results and understanding the experimental parameters, Carrel proclaimed that "the cell was immortal."

By examining the health status of the average North American, we have been made painfully aware that there is a nutritional component that is missing from our diets. Factors such as cooking (enzyme denaturing), fertilizers,

---

[43] Fletcher R H, Fairfield K M. Vitamins for chronic disease prevention in adults: scientific review. *JAMA*. 2002; 287(23):p3116-26.
[44] Vellas B J, Albarede J L, Garry P J. Diseases and aging: patterns of morbidity and age; relationship between aging and age associated diseases. *Am J Clin Nutr*. 1992; 55:p1225S-1230S.
[45] Alexis Carrel. The Columbia Electronic Encyclopedia, 6th ed. Copyright 2007, Columbia University Press.
<http://www.infoplease.com/ce6/people/A0810580.html>.
[46] Lindsten J, Ed. Nobel Lectures, Physiology or Medicine 1901-1921. Elsevier Publishing Company. Amsterdam. 1967.

pesticides, preservatives, chilling, storage and reheating that could affect the bioavailability of nutrients[47] and their subsequent absorption are, potentially impairing physiological function. There is nutrition in our food, although it is affected by a number of factors, and our body's function is improved and maintained by these nutrients. It would really help if we could supplement our diets with a bioavailable superfood.

The advances of technology such as genetic modification of plants, mechanized processing, storage, and shipping modes, in conjunction with faster paced lifestyles, have altered our dietary patterns to the point where most of us are not ingesting the basic minimum nutrition. This protocol is exposing more than half of the population to nutrient related disease risk. The correlation between nutrition and many of the chronic diseases exists and one does not have to have a deficiency status to be affected, only a sub-optimal intake.

A great deal of investigation has gone into the aging process with the concomitant chronic disease and antioxidants have been a focal point. Free radical damage caused by electron-seeking, highly reactive, oxidative molecules has been identified as the source of these maladies. The body, and most of the universe for that matter, is composed predominantly of hydrogen. Most of the reactions that occur in our bodies are related to hydrogen, either as a catalyst, reagent or electron donor[48]. When we are born our bodies have a negative electrical charge, due in a large part to our negatively charged hydrogen stores. As we age, our hydrogen stores are depleted due to the multiple functions hydrogen serves, and unless they are restored, the free radicals will start to act on

---

[47]Fairfield K M, Fletcher R H. Vitamins for chronic disease prevention in adults: scientific review. *JAMA*. 2002; 287(23):p3116-3126.
[48] Lehninger AL, Nelson DL, Cox MM. Bioenergetics and metabolism. In Principles of biochemistry 2nd ed. New York. Worth Publishing. 1993.

body structures such as cell walls and DNA. All of the amino acids of DNA are joined by hydrogen bonds and a powerful enough free radical can pull a hydrogen electron away from a DNA molecule rendering it imperfect. If the body happens to call upon that unit of DNA to reproduce, it may do so imperfectly, due to damaged genetic material. When a cell, or group of cells, proliferate inappropriately, it is called cancer. Curiously all cancer cells are devoid of hydrogen and unable to proliferate in an alkaline medium.

So what can be done? We have all heard of anti-oxidants. Anti-oxidants are substances that are generally ingested and provide electrons to bind with dangerous free radicals and neutralize them in order for the body to dispose of them. If there were a method by which countless negatively charged ions could be delivered into our body (most of us aren't getting it from our cooked processed food diets anymore) would it not be totally beneficial? In the recent past, everyone was scrambling to find powerful anti-oxidants. The cause of aging, along with most of humanity's diseases, has been determined to be due, in large part, to actions of free radicals on our body. Antioxidants such as vitamins A, C, E and selenium will release an electron to a free radical and bind it, transforming it into a relatively harmless molecule fit for excretion. Incidentally, vitamins A, C, E and selenium are all found in Moringa.[49][50][51]

The sources of these free radicals come from both inside the body and the external environment.

[49] Babu S C. Rural nutrition interventions with indigenous plant foods: a case study of vitamin deficiency in Malawi. International Food Policy Research Institute, Washington, DC. *Biotechnology, Agronomy Soc. Environ.* 2000 ;4(3):p.169-179.

[50] Delisle H, Bakari S, et al. Provitamin A content of traditional green leaves from Niger. *Cahiers Agricultures* 1997;6(6):p,553-560.

[51] Fahey J W. *Moringa oleifera*: a review of the medical evidence for its nutritional, therapeutic, and prophylactic properties. *Trees for Life Journal.* 2005;1(5) p. 1-13.

Mitochondria generate the reactive oxygen species as a function of creating ATP and reducing oxygen. Toxic chemicals and ionizing radiation are other prominent sources of free radicals. These oxidants promote aging by attacking lipids in cellular membranes causing increased membrane rigidity, dysfunctional permeability and decreased activity of membrane receptors. Furthermore, membrane proteins,[52] including DNA,[53] will be attacked causing aberrant physiological function and potential cross-linking. Free radicals also inhibit the production of telomerase as we shall discuss later.

Although there are many endogenous antioxidants, it is imperative to ingest dietary antioxidants to minimize the aging process damage caused by free radicals. Several researchers such as Ganguly (2006), Ashok (2003) and Kumar (2003) have determined that Moringa is an excellent source of multiple antioxidants and these findings have been cited by many other authors as well.[54 55 56 57 58 59 60 61 62 63]

[52] Schafer F Q, Wang H P, Kelley E E, Cuenko K L et al. Comparing beta-carotene, vitamin E and nitric oxide as membrane antioxidants. *Biological Chemistry*. 2002; 383:p671-681.
[53] Sies H, Menck C F. Singlet oxygen induced DNA damage. *Mutation Research*. 1992; 275:p367-375.
[54] Ganguly R, Guha D. Protective role of an Indian herb, Moringa oleifera in memory impairment by high altitude hypoxic exposure: Possible role of monoamines. *Biogenic Amines*. 2006;20:p.121-33.
[55] Holst S. *Moringa: Nature's Medicine Cabinet*. Sierra Sunrise Publishing, Sherman Oaks, CA. 2000.128 pp.
[56] Kumar N A, Pari I. Antioxidant action of Moringa oleifera Lam (drumstick) against antitubercular drug induced lipid peroxidation in rats. *J Medicinal Foods*. 2003;6(3):p.255-259.
[57] Bharali R, Tabassum J, Azad M R H. Chemomodulatory effect of *Moringa oleifera*, Lam, on hepatic carcinogen metabolizing enzymes, antioxidant parameters and skin papillomagenesis in mice. *Asian Pacific Journal of Cancer Prevention* 2003;4:p.131-139.
[58] Njoku O U, Adikwu M U. Investigation on some physico-chemical antioxidant and toxicological properties of *Moringa oleifera* seed oil. *Acta Pharmaceutica Zagreb*. 1997;47(4): p.87-290.
[59] Siddhuraju P, Becker K. Antioxidant properties of various solvent extracts of total phenolic constituents from three different agroclimatic

immune, endocrine and neurological systems causing almost any disorder.

The significance of the NHATS study is that it demonstrates that we have all been affected by environmental toxicity. It may seem more severe now, but the problems have been around for a long time, and the toxins are perseverant. DDT (dichloro-diphenyltrichloroethane) was perhaps the most widely used pesticide on the planet, however the use of DDT was banned in the United States in 1972.[28] DDE and DDD are similar chemicals to DDT and were often found to contaminate commercial preparations of DDT. DDD is a banned pesticide itself but DDE is a breakdown product of DDT. DDE was found in the fat of 93% of the population.

Across the border to the north, a combination of harmful toxins has been found inside every person tested in a Canada-wide study, released by a concerned consumer organization, Environmental Defense. The blood and urine of eleven volunteers were tested ranging from British Columbia to Newfoundland (coast to coast) looking for the presence of eighty-eight (88) different chemical toxins. Toxic chemicals, such as DDT, PCBs, stain repellants, flame retardants, mercury and lead, were found to be contaminating Canadians. Many of the chemicals are associated with cancer, hormone disruption, reproductive disorders, respiratory illnesses and harming the development of children. Most exposure to these three xenobiotics occurs through ingestion of food and beverage. It appears to be endemic in our ecosystems and yet it can be demonstrated in fat, blood, urine, semen and breast milk. It has been more

---

[28] Agency for Toxic Substances and Disease Registry (ATSDR). *Toxilogical Profile for DDT, DDE, and DDD. Update.* Atlanta, GA. U.S. Department of Health and Human Services, Public Health Service. 2002.
[29] Haas, Elson M. Staying Healthy With Nutrition: The Complete Guide to Diet and Nutritional Medicine. Berkeley, California. Celestial Arts. 1992. p906.

Researchers have been trying to determine the necessary nutrients that the body needs for optimal health and the best methods for not only their bioavailability, but subsequent absorption after ingestion and maximal physiological utilization. The facts are clear: if you ingest fruit, vegetables and/or nutritional supplements, your serum levels of vitamins, minerals and trace elements will be higher,[64] [65] and this will confer a protective element against chronic diseases.[66] [67] This knowledge will allow an individual to formulate a nutritional plan of action and include *Moringa oleifera*

origins of drumstick tree (*Moringa oleifera* Lam.) leaves. *Journal of Agricultural and Food Chemistry*. 2003;51:p.2144-2155.
[60] Fahey J W, Dinkova-Kostova A T, Talalay P. *The "Prochaska" microtiter plate bioassay for inducers of NQO1*. Chapter 14 in Methods in Enzymology, Vol. 382, Part B, 2004;p. 243-258 (Eds.) H. Sies & L. Packer, Elsevier Science, San Diego, CA. 2004.
[61] Faizi S, Siddiqui B S, Saleem R, Aftab K, Shaheen F, Gilani A H. Bioactive Compounds from the leaves and pods of *Moringa oleifera*. *New Trends in Natural Products Chemistry* 1998;p.175-183.
[62] Rao K N V, Gopalakrishnan V, Loganathan V, Shanmuganathan S. Antiinflammatory activity of *Moringa oleifera* Lam. *Ancient Science of Life* 1999;18(3-4):p.195-198.
[63] Ashok K, Pari, L. Antioxidant action of Moringa oleifera Lam. (drumstick) against antitubercular drugs induced lipid peroxidation in rats. J Med Food. 2003; Fall; 6 (3):p.255-9.
[64] Mckay D L, Perrone G, Rasmussen H, Dallal G, et al. The effects of a multivitamin/mineral supplement on micronutrient status, antioxidant capacity and cytokine production in healthy older adults consuming a fortified diet. *J Am Coll Nutr*. 2000; 19(5):p613-621.
[65] Preziosi P, Galan P, Herbeth B, Valeix P, et al. Effects of supplementation with a combination of antioxidant vitamins and trace elements at nutritional doses, on biochemical indicators and markers of the antioxidant system in adult subjects. *J Am Coll Nutr*. 1998; 17(3):p244-249.
[66] Block G, Patterson B, Subar A. Fruit, vegetables, and cancer prevention: a review of the epidemiological evidence. *Nutr Cancer*. 1992; 18:p1-29.
[67] Steinmetz K A, Potter J D. Vegetables, fruit, and cancer protection: a review. *J Am Diet Assoc*. 1996: 96:p1027-1039.

Epidemiological findings and investigative research
advocate a direct relationship between nutrition, diet and
chronic diseases.[68] [69] [70] [71] [72] Another aspect of health that
has an overriding effect on all disease is the status of the
immune system.   Approximately 98% of the North
American population has a diminished immune function.[73]

The correlation between nutrition and immune
system enhancement is well documented in the review of
scientific literature.[74] [75] [76] [77] [78] More direct randomized

[68] Herder R, Demmig-Adams B. The power of a balanced diet and
lifestyle in preventing cardiovascular disease. *Nutr Clin Care*. 2004;
7(2):46-55.
[69] Gaziano J M, Manson J E. Diet and heart disease. The role of fat,
alcohol, and antioxidants. *Cardiol Clin*. 1996; 14(1):p69-83.
[70] Eyre H, Kahn, R, Robertson R M. American Cancer Society,
American Diabetes Association, and American Heart Association
Collaborative Writing Committees. Preventing Cancer, cardiovascular
disease, and diabetes: a common agenda for the American Cancer
Society, the American Diabetes Association, and the American Heart
Association. *Diabetes Care*. 2004; 27(7):p1812-24.
[71] Donaldson M S. Nutrition and Cancer: A review of the evidence for
an anti-cancer diet. *Nutrition Journal*. 2004; 3(19).
[72] Key T J, Schatzkin A, Willett W C, Allen N E, Spencer E A et al.
Diet, nutrition, and the prevention of cancer. *Public Health Nutr*.
2004; 7(1A):p187-200.
[73] Stoff J. An Examination of Immune Response Modulation in
Humans by Antigen Infused Dialyzable Bovine Colostrum/Whey
Extract Using A Double Blind Study. Tucson. Immune Consultants.
2001.
[74] Chandra R K. Effect of vitamin and trace-element supplementation
on immune responses and infection in elderly subjects. *Lancet*. 1992;
340:p1124-7.
[75] Fawzi W, Stanpfer MJ. A role for multivitamins in infection? *Ann
Int Med*. 2003; 138(5):p430-431.
[76] Meydani S N, Meydani M, Blumberg J B, et al. Vitamin E
supplementation and in vivo immune response in healthy elderly
subjects: a randomized controlled trial. *JAMA*. 1997; 277:p1380-1386.
[77] Chandra R K. Nutrition and the immune system from birth to old
age. *Eur J Clin Nutr*. 2002; 131:p2192-2196.
[78] Chandra R K. Influence of multinutrient supplement on immune
responses and infection-related illness in 50-65 year old individuals.
Nutr Res. 2002; 22:p5-11.

clinical trials are necessary to sort out all of the individual components, but the facts remain that our bodies require certain nutrients: water, vitamins, minerals, and antioxidants to function at an optimal level. Somehow we have overlooked this information in our quest for creature comforts and technological advancement. We are approaching the time when technological advancement can reflect upon our pending nutritional crisis. The bulk of the population is aging and being subjected, possibly quite unnecessarily, to many chronic diseases and concomitant immune system dysfunction related to nutritional shortfalls. This niche is exactly where *Moringa oleifera* fits in as a vehicle to change the health profile.

The current multi-billion dollar supplement industry would not sustain the substantial growth it is currently enjoying if there were no reason to supplement, and if people were not deriving benefits. Of course the question must be asked about the reasons that we can no longer derive adequate nutrition from our food supply.

By definition alone, the word supplement means to replace that which is missing and that in fact should be the key to the answer. We have known for over half a century that our food sources have been deficient in vitamins and minerals.[79] Harvesting and shipping modes do not take nutrition into account and in combination with extensive processing, improper storage and soil deficiencies, it is almost impossible to get adequate nutrition from our current food supply.[80] There is a great deal of evidence supporting supplementation and the consequent decreased risk of diseases. According to the Council for Responsible Nutrition, "There is ample evidence to suggest that the public will benefit from the adoption of healthy dietary

---

[79] Beach R. Modern Miracle Men. Washington. United States Government Printing Office Document No. 264. 1941.
[80] Balch J, Balch P. Prescription for Nutritional Healing. New York. Avery Publishing Group. 2000; p14.

patterns and healthy lifestyle habits including the regular use of nutritional supplements."[81] "Antioxidants have long been linked to the prevention of degenerative diseases associated with aging,"[82] and Moringa is rich in antioxidants such as vitamin A, vitamin C, selenium, and vitamin E.[83] [84] A review of the literature concerning the relationship between nutrition and disease confirms the need for something more than the average diet is currently providing.[85]

CANCER

According to nationally renowned Oncologist and Immunologist, Dr. Charles B. Simone, "Nutritional deficiencies decrease a person's capacity to resist infection and its consequences and decrease the capability of the immune system."[86] When we combine that information with, "protective elements in a cancer prevention diet that include selenium, folic acid, vitamin B-12, vitamin D, chlorophyll, and antioxidants such as the carotenoids (alpha carotene, beta carotene, lycopene, lutein, cryptoxanthin,"[87] it becomes obvious that intelligent use of nutrients can, in fact, affect chronic disease. Carotenoids such as beta-

[81] Dickinson A, Ed. The Benefits of Nutritional Supplements. Washington. Council for Responsible Nutrition. 1998; p61.
[82] Hallfrisch J H, Muller D C, Singh D M. Vitamin A and E intake plasma concentration of retinol, beta.carotene, alpha-tocophero in men and women of the Baltimore longitudinal study of aging. *Am J Clin Nutr*. 1992; 1994; 60:p176-182.
[83] Fuglie L J. *The Miracle Tree: Moringa oleifera: Natural Nutrition for the Tropics*. Church World Service, Dakar. 1999;68 pp.
[84] Njoku O U, Adikwu M U. Investigation on some physico-chemical antioxidant and toxicological properties of *Moringa oleifera* seed oil. *Acta Pharmaceutica Zagreb*. 1997;47(4):p.87-290.
[85]Fletcher R H, Fairfield K M. Vitamins for chronic disease prevention in adults: scientific review. *JAMA*. 2002; 287(23):p3116-26.
[86] Simone C. Cancer and Nutrition. Garden City Park, New York. Avery Publishing Group. 1992; p46.
[87] Donaldson M S. Nutrition and Cancer: A review of the evidence for an anti-cancer diet. *Nutrition Journal*. 2004; 3(19).

carotene, lycopene, zeaxanthin, and lutein have been singled out for their benefits on decreasing total cancer risk and prostate cancer risk specifically.[88 89 90 91 92 93 94 95 96 97 98 99 100 101 102 103 104]

[88] Christen W G, Gaziano M, Hennekens C H. Design of Physicians' Health Study II- A Randomized Trial of Beta-Carotene, Vitamins E and C, and Multivitamins, in Prevention of Cancer, Cardiovascular Disease, and Eye Disease, and Review of Results of Completed Trials. *Annals of Epidemiology*. 2000; 10(2):p125-134

[89] Deming D M, Boileau T, Heintz K H, Arkinson C A, Erdman J W Jr. Carotenoids: Linking chemistry, absorption, and metabolism to potential roles in human health and disease. In Cadenas E, and Packer L, (Eds). Handbook of Antioxidants. Marcel-Dekker. New York. 2002; p189-221.

[90]Giovannucci E, Stampfer M J, Colditz G A, Hunter D J, Fuchs C, et al. Multivitamin use, folate and colon cancer in women in the Nurses' Health Study. *Ann Intern Med*. 1998; 129(7):p517-24.

[91] Giovannucci E, Ascherio A, Rimm E B, Stampfer M J, Colditz G A, Willett W. Intake of carotenoids and retinol in relation to risk of prostate cancer. *J Natl Cancer Inst*. 1995; 87: p1767-1776.

[92] Giovannucci E, Rimm E B, Stampfer M J, Willett W. A prospective study of tomato products, lycopene and prostate cancer risk.. *J Natl Cancer Inst*. 2002; 94: p391-398.

[93] Chan J M, Stampfer M J, Ma J, Rimm E B, Willett W C, Giovannucci E L. Supplemental Vitamin E intake and prostate cancer risk in a large cohort of men in the United States. *Cancer Epidemiol Biomarkers Prev*. 1999; 8:p893-899.

[94] Alpha-Tocopherol Beta-Carotene Cancer Prevention Study Group. The effect of vitamin E and beta carotene on the incidence of lung cancer and other cancers in male smokers, *N Engl J Med*. 1994; 330:p1029-1035.

[95] Speizer F E, Colditz G A, Hunter D J, Rosner B, et al. Prospective study of smoking, antioxidant intake, and lung cancer in middle-aged women (USA). *Cancer Causes Control*. 1999; 10:p475-482.

[96] Michaud D S, Feskanich D, Rimm E B, et al. Intake of specific carotenoids and the risk of lung cancer in 2 prospective US cohorts. *Am J Clin Nutr*. 2000; 72:p990-997.

[97] Hsing A W, Comstock G W, Abbey H, Polk B F. Serologic precursors of cancer. Retinol, carotenoids and tocopherol and risk of prostate cancer. *J Natl Cancer Inst*. 1990; 82:p941-946.

[98] Knekt P, Jarvinen, Teppo L, Aromaa A, Seppanen R. Role of various carotenoids in lung cancer prevention. *J Natl Cancer Inst*. 1999; 91:p182-184.

One interesting difference in the nature of the carotenoid antioxidants is in the way they scavenge free radicals. Carotenoids are usually found in colorful red, orange and yellow plants and there are more than six hundred, many of which are retinol precursors. Most antioxidants give up an electron to satiate the free radical before it can damage collagen, cell walls or DNA. The free radicals then enter the electron cascade and seek another electron from some other antioxidant to replenish itself and subsequently seek another free radical.

Carotenoids function in a different manner. They will scavenge fifteen to twenty free radicals and then degenerate, not entering the electron cascade and acting as a less vigorous free radical, similar to other antioxidants. This makes them a vital component to the body's antioxidant system. Carotenoids are exceptional scavengers of oxygen singlet free radicals[105] and with the predisposition of these antagonists to attack cellular

[99] Cook N R, Stampfer M J, Ma J, et al. Beta-carotene supplementation for patients with low baseline levels and decreased risks of total and prostate carcinoma. *Cancer*. 1999; 86:p1783-1792.
[100] Zhang S, Hunter D J, Forman M R, et al. Dietary carotenoids and vitamins A, C, E and risk of breast cancer. *J Natl Cancer Inst*. 1999; 91:p547-556.
[101] Schuurman A G, Goldbohm R A, Brants H A, van den Brandt P A. A prospective cohort study on intake of retinol, vitamins C and E, and carotenoids and prostate cancer risk (Netherlands). *Cancer Causes Control*. 2002; 13:p573-582.
[102] Wu K, Erdman J W Jr, Schwartz S J, Platz E A, Leitzmann M, et al. Plasma and dietary carotenoids, and the risk of prostate cancer: a nested case-control study. *Cancer Epidemiol Biomarkers Prev*. 2004; 13:p260-269.
[103] Kucuk O, Sarkar F H, Sakr W, Djuric Z,Pollak M N, et al. Phase II randomized clinical trial of lycopene supplementation before radical prostatectomy. *Cancer Epidemiol Biomarkers Prev*. 2001; 10:p886-893.
[104] Giles G, Ireland P. Diet, nutrition and prostate cancer. *Int J Cancer*. 1997; 72:p13-17.
[105] Di Mascio p, Murphy M E, Sies H. Antioxidant defense systems: The role of carotenoids, tocopherols and thiols. *Am J Clin Nutr*. 1991; 53:p194S-200S.

membranes, they demonstrate a high degree of protection for cellular integrity.[106]

Carotenoid levels can serve as a direct reflection of dietary intake of fruits and vegetables and antioxidant supplements. "Skin carotenoid levels correlate well with blood carotenoid levels and may more accurately indicate carotenoid status, because, unlike blood, skin carotenoids are not influenced by postprandial fluctuations."[107]

Moringa has been shown to be rich in antioxidant carotenoids such as beta-carotene and provitamin A. Delisle (1997), Nambiar (2001) and Subadra (1997) have confirmed this fact.[108] [109] [110] There is a lot of research indicating that there are many other phytonutrients in Moringa that combat cancer.[111] [112] [113] [114] [115] [116] [117] [118] [119] [120] [121] [122] [123]

[106] Smidt C R, Burke D S. Nutritional significance and measurement of carotenoids. *Current Topics in Nutritional Research.* 2004; 2(2):p79-91

[107] Smidt C R, Burke D S. Nutritional significance and measurement of carotenoids. *Current Topics in Nutritional Research.* 2004; 2(2):p79-91.

[108] Delisle H, Bakari S, et al. Provitamin A content of traditional green leaves from Niger. *Cahiers Agricultures* 1997;6(6):p,553-560

[109] Nambiar V S, Seshadri S. Bioavailability trials of beta-carotene from fresh and dehydrated leaves of *Moringa oleifera* in a rat model. *Plant Foods for Human Nutrition.* 2001;56(1): 83-95.

[110] Subadra S, Monica J et al. Retention and storage stability of beta-carotene in dehydrated drumstick leaves (*Moringa oleifera*) *Int J Food Sciences and Nutrition.* 1997;48(6):p.373-379.

[111] Jayavardhanan K K, K Suresh K, Panikkar K R, Vasudevan D M. Modulatory potency of drumstick lectin on the host defense system. *Journal of Experimental Clinical Cancer Research* 1994;13(3):p.205-209.

[112] Hartwell J L. Plants used against cancer: a survey. *Lloydia* 1971;p.30-34.

[113] Gupta M, UK Mazumder U K, et al. Anti-epileptic and anti-cancer activity of some indigenous plants. *Indian Journal of Physiology and Allied Sciences* 1997;51(2):p.53-56.

Isothiocyanates battle carcinogens by neutralizing them: inhibiting cellular proliferation and causing apoptosis in the cancer cells (cell death). Furthermore, isothiocyanates act to prevent certain cancers: lung, esophageal, and gastrointestinal. Moringa contains

[114] Faizi S, Siddiqui B S, Saleem R, Aftab K, Shaheen F, Gilani A H. Bioactive Compounds from the leaves and pods of *Moringa oleifera*. *New Trends in Natural Products Chemistry* 1998;p.175-183.
[115] Fahey J W, Dinkova-Kostova A T, Talalay P. *The "Prochaska" microtiter plate bioassay for inducers of NQO1*. Chapter 14 in Methods in Enzymology, Vol. 382, Part B, 2004;p. 243-258 (Eds.) H. Sies & L. Packer, Elsevier Science, San Diego, CA. 2004.
[116] Fahey J W, Haristoy X, Dolan P M, Kensler T W, Scholtus I, Stephenson K K, Talalay P, Lozniewski A. (2002) Sulforaphane inhibits extracellular, intracellular, and antibiotic-resistant strains of *Helicobacter pylori* and prevents benzo[*a*]pyrene-induced stomach tumors. *Proceedings of the National Academy of Sciences USA* 2002;99:p.7610-7615.
[117] Delaveau P, et al. (1980) Oils of *Moringa oleifera* and *Moringa drouhardii*. *Plantes Médicinales et Phytothérapie* 1980;14(10):p.29-33.
[118] Costa-Lotufo LV, Khan M T H, Ather A, Wilke D V, Jimenez P C, Pessoa C, MEA de Moraes MO de Moraes (2005) Studies of the anticancer potential of plants used in Bangladeshi folk medicine. *J Ethnopharmacology* 2005;99: p.21-30.
[119] Bharali R, Tabassum J, Azad M R H. Chemomodulatory effect of *Moringa oleifera*, Lam, on hepatic carcinogen metabolizing enzymes, antioxidant parameters and skin papillomagenesis in mice. *Asian Pacific Journal of Cancer Prevention* 2003;4:p.131-139.
[120] Bennett R N, Mellon F A, Foidl N, Pratt J H, DuPont M S, Perkins L, Kroon P A. Profiling glucosinolates and phenolics in vegetative and reproductive tissues of the multi-purpose trees *Moringa oleifera* L. (Horseradish tree) and *Moringa stenopetala* L. *J Agricultural and Food Chemistry*. 2003;51: p.3546-3553.
[121] Jadhav S L, Sharma S R, Pal S C, Kasture S B, Kasture V S. (2000) Chemistry and pharmacology of *Moringa oleifera* and *Moringa concanescens* Niro. *Indian Drugs* 2000;37(3):p.139-144.
[122] Pal S K, Mukherjee P K, Saha B P. Studies on the antiulcer activity of *Moringa oleifera* leaf extract on gastric ulcer models in rats. *Phytotherapy Research*. 1995;9:p.463-465.
[123] Fuglie L J. *The Miracle Tree: Moringa oleifera: Natural Nutrition for the Tropics*. Church World Service, Dakar. 1999;68pp.

isothiocyanates.[124] Moringa leaves contain a thiocarbamate, niaziminin.[125] [126] Niaziminin has shown the ability to inhibit a tumor promoter. Naturally far more research is necessary to make medical claims, but the indications reveal that the relationships are already established.

Antioxidants are leading the way in the battle of anti-aging and chronic disease. Anti-oxidants provide an electron to neutralize a free radical and prevent the free radical from causing anatomical damage by removing an electron and degenerating a tissue or DNA molecule. Researchers have known for decades that much of the cellular degeneration that leads to aging and chronic disease is caused by Reactive Oxygen Species (free radicals) that oxidize various parts of the body.[127] [128] [129] [130] [131] [132] [133]

[124] Kjaer A, Malver O, El-Menshawi B, Reisch J. Isothiocyanates in myrosinase-treated seed extracts of *Moringa peregrina*. *Phytochemistry* 1979;18:p.1485-1487.
[125] Murakami A, Kitazono Y, Jiwajinda S, Koshimizu K, Ohigashi H. Niaziminin, a thiocarbamate from the leaves of *Moringa oleifera*, holds a strict structural requirement for inhibition of tumor-promoter-induced Epstein-Barr virus activation. *Planta Medica* 1998;64: p.319-323.
[126] Guevara A P, Vargas C, Sakurai H, Fujiwara Y, Hashimoto K, Maoka T, Kozuka M, Ito Y, Tokuda H, Nishino H. An antitumor promoter from *Moringa oleifera* Lam. *Mutation Research* 1999;440:p.181-188.
[127] Dizdoroglu M, Jaruga P, Birincioglu M, Rodriguez H. Free radical induced damage to DNA: mechanisms and measurement. *Free Radical Biology and Medicine*. 2002; 32:p1102-1115.
[128] Diplock A T. Antioxidant nutrients and disease prevention: an overview. *Am J Clin Nutr*. 1991; 53:p194S-200S.
[129] Wickens A P. Ageing and the free radical theory. *Respiration Physiology*. 2001; 128:p379-391.
[130] Moskovitz J, Yim M B, Chock P B. Free radicals and disease. *Archives of Biochemistry and Biophysics*. 2002; 397:p354-359.
[131] Hensley K, Floyd R A. Reactive oxygen species and protein oxidation in aging: A look back, a look ahead. *Archives of Biochemistry and Biophysics*. 2002; 397:p373-383.
[132] Schafer F Q, Wang H P, Kelley E E, Cuenko K L et al. Comparing beta-carotene, vitamin E and nitric oxide as membrane antioxidants. *Biological Chemistry*. 2002; 383:p671-681.

We cannot avoid these free radicals. Aside from the fact that we come in contact with billions of the electron seeking molecules daily from external sources and pollutants, every mitochondrion in every cell produces them as a by-product of energy (ATP) production. Science has progressed to the point that availability of antioxidants will allow the body to eliminate the damage caused by free radicals (oxidative stress). The relationship between telomeres, aging and disease was recently brought to light by Blackburn et al (2006).[134] She and her co-authors were awarded the Nobel Prize in Physiology and Medicine in 2009 for their discovery of the protective cap at the end of chromosomes, telomeres. They shorten every time a cell divides and when they become too short, the cell can no longer divide and the cell dies.[135] The pace at which telomeres shorten is associated with the cell's ability to withstand oxidative damage,[136] therefore the more antioxidants present in one's body, the less damage that occurs to the chromosome.[137]

The Agricultural Research Service's Human Nutrition Research Center on Aging at Tufts suggests that diets containing fruits and vegetables with high antioxidant potential may help to slow down the aging process and

---

[133] Sohal R S, Mockett R J, Orr W C. Mechanisms of aging: An appraisal of the oxidative stress hypothesis. *Free Radical Biology and Medicine*. 2002; 33:p575-586.
[134] Blackburn et al. Telomeres and telomerase: The path from maize, *Tetrahymena* and yeast to human cancer and aging. *Nature Medicine*. 2006;12:p.1133-1138.
[135] Allsopp R C, Harley C B, Evidence for a critical telomere length in senescent human fibroblasts. *Experimental Cell Res*. 1995;219:p.130-136.
[136] Sozou P D, Kirkwood T B. A stochastic model of cell replicative senescence based on telomere shortening,oxidative stress, and somatic mutations in nuclear and mitochondrial DNA. *J Theoretical Biology*.2001;213:p.573-576.
[137] Serra V, Grune T, Sitte N, Saretzki G, von Zglinicki T. Telomere length as a marker of oxidative stress in primary human fibroblast cultures. *Annals of the New York Academy of Sciences*. 2000;908:p.327-330.

therefore affect chronic disease,[138] and certainly the
Moringa family of plants demonstrate significant
antioxidant levels.

Other antioxidants, such as vitamin C and vitamin
E, have also been linked to a reduction in cancer risk.[139] [140]
[141] [142] [143] [144] Well known Moringa researcher, Lowell Fuglie
has related the fact that the miracle tree has significantly
more vitamin C then a highly popular vitamin C source-
oranges.[145] [146] Other researchers concur with the
disproportionate amount of Vitamin C and other vitamins
and minerals present in Moringa, citing that less than one
ounce of Moringa leaf powder provides forty-two percent
(42%) of the recommended daily allowance of protein,
more than all of the calcium requirements, sixty-one
percent (61%) of the magnesium, forty-one percent (41%)
of recommended potassium, almost triple the vitamin A

---

[138] Gaziano J M, Manson J E, Branch L G, Colditz G A, et al. A
prospective study of consumption of carotenoids in fruits and
vegetables and decreased cardiovascular mortality in the elderly. *Ann
Epidemol_1995; 5:p 225*
[139] Jacobs E J, Connell C J, Patel A C, Chao A, et al. Multivitamin use
and colon cancer mortality in the Cancer Prevention Study II cohort
(United States). *Cancer Causes Control.* 2001; 12(10):p.927-934.
[140] Byers T, Guerrero N. Epidemiologic evidence for vitamin C and
vitamin E in cancer prevention. *Am J Clin Nutr.* 1995; 62:p1385S-
1392S.
[141] Negri E, Franceschi S, Bosetti C, et al. Selected micronutrients and
oral and pharyngeal cancer. *Int J Cancer.* 2000; 86:p122-127.
[142] You W C, Zhang L, Gail M H, et al. Gastric dysplasia and gastric
cancer: Helicobacter pylori, serum vitamin C, and other risk factors. *J
Natl Cancer Inst.* 2000; 92:p1607-1612.
[143] Gandini S, Merzenich H, Robertson C, Boyle P. Meta-analysis of
studies on breast cancer risk and diet: the role of fruit and vegetable
consumption and the intake of associated micronutirents. *Eur J
Cancer.* 2000; 36:p636-646.
[144] Lee K W, Lee H J, Surh Y J, Lee C Y. Vitamin C and cancer
chemoprevention: reappraisal. *Am J Clin Nutr.* 2003; 78: p1074-1078.
[145] Fuglie L J. *The Miracle Tree: Moringa oleifera: Natural Nutrition
for the Tropics.* Church World Service, Dakar. 1999;68pp.
[146] Fuglie L J. New uses of Moringa studied in Nicaragua. ECHO
Development Notes #68, June, 2000.

(272%), seventy-one percent (71%) of the iron and twenty-two percent (22%) of the RDA for Vitamin C.[147]

There are many other nutrients that have been shown to decrease cancer risk, that are generally considered to be part of a basic vitamin regimen such as folate,[148] vitamin B12,[149][150] and vitamin D,[151] to name a few.

CARDIOVASCULAR DISEASE

Cardiovascular disease is still the number one killer on the planet, and according to the World Health Organization causing or contributing to more than 13 million deaths between heart disease, cerebrovascular disease and stroke.[152] It is a well documented fact that fruit and vegetable consumption provides a protective relationship for heart disease, myocardial infarct and ischemic stroke (CVD). [153][154] Researchers, such as Dr.

---

[147] Ramachandran C, Peter K V, Gopalakrishnan P K. 1980, Drumstick (Moringa oleifera): A multipurpose Indian Vegetable. *Economic Botany*, 34 (3) p.276-283.

[148] Kim Y I. Folate and cancer prevention: a new medical application of folate beyond hyperhomocysteinemia and neural tube defects. *Nutr Rev.* 1999; 57:p314-321.

[149] Wu K, Helzlsouer K J, Comstock G W, Hoffman S C, Nadeau M R, Selhub J, Mason J B. A prospective study on folate, B12, and pyridoxal 5'-phosphate (B6) and breast cancer. *Cancer Epidemiol Biomarkers Prev.* 1999; 8:p209-217.

[150] Zhang S M, Willet W C, Selhub J, Hunter D J, Giovannucci E L, Holmes M D, Colditz G A, Hankinson S E. Plasma folate, B6, vitamin B12, homocysteine, and risk of breast cancer. *J Natl Cancer Inst.* 2003; 95:p373-380.

[151] Hollick M F, Vitamin D: importance in the prevention of cancers, type 1 diabetes, heart disease and osteoporosis. *Am J Clin Nutr.* 2004; 79:p362-371.

[152] http://www.who.int/mediacentre/factsheets/fs310/en/index.html

[153] Joshipura K J, Ascherio A, Manson J E, et al. Fruit and vegetable intake in relation to risk of ischemic stroke. *JAMA.* 1999; 282:p1233-1239.

[154] Joshipura K J, Hu F B, Manson J E, et al. The effect of fruit and vegetable intake on risk for coronary heart disease. *Ann Intern Med.* 2001; 134:p1106-1114.

Joshipura and many others, acknowledge that this protective effect can be explained by nutritional components in the fruit such as vitamins, folate, potassium, antioxidants, [155] [156] [157] [158] [159] and fiber. [160] [161] The recommended dosage is more than five servings of fruits and vegetables daily,[162] or the commensurate amount of nutrient supplementation. The Moringaceae are capable of providing these phytonutrients.[163] [164] [165]

[155] Knekt P, Reunanen A, Jarvinen R, Seppanen R, et al. Antioxidant vitamin intake and coronary mortality in a longitudinal population study. *Am J Epidemiol.* 1994; 139:p1180-1189.
[156] Hodis H N, Mack W J, LaBree L, et al. Serial coronary angiographic evidence that antioxidant vitamin intake reduces progression of coronary artery atherosclerosis. *JAMA.* 1995; 273: p1849-1854.
[157] Rimm E B, Willet W C, Hu F B, et al. Folate and Vitamin B6 from diet and supplements in relation to risk of coronary heart disease among women. *JAMA.* 1998; 279:p.359-364.
[158] Evans R W, Shaten B J, Day B W, Kuller L H. Prospective association between lipid soluble antioxidants and coronary heart disease in men: the Multiple Risk Factor Intervention Trial. *Am J Epidemiol.* 1998; 147:p180-186.
[159] Kushi L H, Folsom A R, Prineas R J, Mink P J, et al. Dietary antioxidant vitamins and death from coronary heart disease in postmenopausal women. *N Eng J Med.* 1996; 334(18):p1156-1162.
[160] Rimm E B, Stampfer M J, Ascherio A, et al. Vitamin E consumption and the risk of coronary heart disease in men. *N Engl J Med.* 1993; 328:p1450-1456.
[161] Ward M, McNulty H, McPartlin J, Strain J J, et al. Plasma homocysteine, a risk factor for cardiovascular disease is lowered by physiological doses of folic acid. *QJM.* 1997; 90:p519-524.
[162] Committee on Diet and Health. Diet and Health: Implications for Reducing Chronic Disease Risk. Washington DC. National Academy Press. 1989.
[163] Fuglie L J. *The Miracle Tree: Moringa oleifera: Natural Nutrition for the Tropics.* Church World Service, Dakar. 1999;68pp.
[164] Fahey J W. *Moringa oleifera*: a review of the medical evidence for its nutritional, therapeutic, and prophylactic properties. *Trees for Life Journal.* 2005;1(5) p. 1-13.
[165] Geervani P, Devi A. Influence of protein and fat on the utilisation of carotene from drumstick (*Moringa oleifera*) leaves. *Indian J Med Res.* 1981;74:p.548-553.

A well stated consensus of opinion on the relationship between nutrition and cardiovascular disease (CAD) may be summed up by the statement in the Lewin Group report, "Mild to moderate deficiencies in antioxidant nutrients such as vitamin C, vitamin E and beta-carotene, as well as folic acid, although not severe enough to cause classic deficiency diseases, may be involved in the development of CAD."[166] [167]

The relationship of elevated serum homocysteine as a major risk criterion for CAD has been well documented.[168] [169] [170] [171] Vitamins B6, B12 and folate are needed to convert homocysteine to methionine, however it is the amount of folate that enables this reaction to occur and is thus the reactive determining substance.[172] [173]

---

[166] Dobson A, DaVanzo J, Consunji M, Gilani J, et al. A Study of the Cost Effects of Daily Multivitamins for Older Adults. The Lewin Group. Falls Church, VA. 2004.
[167] Selhub J, Jacques P F, Rosenberg I H et al. Serum total homocysteine concentrations in the third National Health and Nutrition Examination Survey (1991-1994); population reference ranges and contribution of vitamin status to high serum concentrations. *Ann Intern Med.* 1999; 131: p331-339.
[168] Eikelboom J W, Lonn E, Genest J Jr, Hankey G, Yusuf S. Homocysteine and cardiovascular disease: a critical review of the epidemiological evidence. *Ann Intern Med.* 1999; 131:p363-375.
[169] Graham I M, Daly L E, Refsum H M, et al. Plasma homocysteine as a risk factor for vascular disease: the European Concerted Action Project. *JAMA.* 1997; 277:p1775-1781.
[170] Welch G N, Loscalzo J. Homocysteine and atherothrombosis. *N Engl J Med.* 1998; 338:p1042-1050.
[171] Robinson K, Arheart K, Refsum H et al for the European COMAC Group. Low circulating folate and vitamin B6 concentrations: risk factors for stroke, peripheral vascular disease, and coronary artery disease. *Circulation.* 1998; 97:p437-443.
[172] Nygard O, Refsum H, Ueland P M, Vollset S E. Major lifestyle determinants of plasma total homocysteine distribution: the Hordaland Homocysteine Study. *Am J Clin Nutr.* 1998; 67:p263-270.
[173] Selhub J, Jacques PF, Rosenberg IH et al. Serum total homocysteine concentrations in the third National Health and Nutrition Examination Survey (1991-1994); population reference ranges and contribution of

A 1999 study found beta-carotene capable of reducing the risk of myocardial infarction, contradicting the findings of some earlier studies,[174] and the beta carotene content of Moringa has already been established. Several investigators have found connections between carotenoids, lycopene and lutein and the risk of heart disease.[175] [176]

There have been many studies associated with Moringa and heart disease and the various cardiovascular parameters such as high blood pressure (hypertension) and elevated cholesterol. Ghasi et al (2000) and several other researchers (Gilani et al 1994, Mehta et al 2003) have found that nutritional components found in the 'drumstick tree' can reduce serum cholesterol.[177] [178] [179] [180] [181] According

---

vitamin status to high serum concentrations. *Ann Intern Med.* 1999; 131: p331-339.

[174] Klipstein-Grobusch K, Geleijnse J M, den Breeijen J H, Boeing H et al. Dietary antioxidants and risk of myocardial infarction in the elderly: the Rotterdam Study. *Am J Clin Nutr.* 1999; 69(2):p261-266.

[175] Sesso H D, Buring J E, Norkus E P, Gaziano J M. Plasma lycopene, other carotenoids and retinol and the risk of cardiovascular disease in women. *Am J Clin Nutr.* 2004; 79:p47-53.

[176] Cardinault N, Gorrand j M, Tyssandier V, Grolier P, et al. Short term supplementation with lutein affects biomarkers of lutein status similarly in young and elderly subjects. *Experimental Gerontology.* 2003; 38:p573-582.

[177] Ghasi S, Nwobodo E, Ofili J O. Hypocholesterolemic effects of crude extract of leaf of *Moringa oleifera* Lam in high-fat diet fed Wistar rats. *J Ethnopharmacology* 2000 ;69(1):p.21-25.

[178] Gilani A H, Aftab K, Suria A, Siddiqui S, Saleem R, Siddiqui B S, Faizi S. Pharmacological studies on hypotensive and spasmolytic activities of pure compounds from *Moringa oleifera. Phytotherapy Research* 1994;8(2):p.87-91.

[179] Mehta L K, Balaraman R, Amin A H, Bafna P A , Gulati O D. (2003) Effect of fruits of *Moringa oleifera* on the lipid profile of normal and hypocholesterolaemic rabbits. *J Ethnopharmacology* 2003;86:p.191-195.

[180] Dahot M U, Memon A R. Properties of *Moringa oleifera* seed lipase. *Pakistan Journal of Scientific and Industrial Research* 1987;30(11):p.832-835.

[181] Chumark P, Khunawat P, Sanvarinda Y, Phornchirasilp S, Morales N P, Phivthong-ngam L, Ratanachamnong P, Srisawat S, Pongrapeeporn K-S. The *in vitro* and *ex vivo* antioxidant properties,

to the Centers for Disease Control, 31.3% of adults in the
United States have high blood pressure, which has
contributed to 326,000 deaths in 2006 and costs about $75
billion for health care services, medications and missed
days of work (2010).[182] There are multiple studies showing
that adding Moringa to your dietary regimen will reduce
blood pressure.[183] [184] 185 186 187 188 189 190 191 192 193

---

hypolipidaemic and antiatherosclerotic activities of water extract of
Moringa oleifera Lam. leaves. *J Ethnopharmacology*. 2008; 116:p.439-
446.
[182] http://www.cdc.gov/bloodpressure/facts.htm
[183] Faizi S, Siddiqui BS, Saleem R, Siddiqui S, Aftab K, Gilani AH.
Fully acetylated carbamates and hypotensive thiocarbamate glycosides
from Moringa oleifera. Phytochemistry 1995;38:957-63.
[184] Tabassum N, Ahmad F. Role of natural herbs in the treatment of
hypertension. 2011;5:p.30-40.
[185] Saleem R, Meinwald J. Synthesis of novel hypotensive aromatic
thiocarbamate glycosides. *Journal of the Chemical Society Perkins
Transactions*. 2000;1: 391-394.
[186] Fuglie L J. *The Miracle Tree: Moringa oleifera: Natural Nutrition
for the Tropics*. Church World Service, Dakar. 1999;68pp.
[187] Faizi S, Siddiqui B S, Saleem R, Aftab K, Shaheen F, Gilani A H.
Hypotensive constituents from the pods of *Moringa oleifera*. *Planta
Medica* 1998;64:p.225-228.
[188] Faizi S, Siddiqui B S, Saleem R, Aftab K, Shaheen F, Gilani A H.
Fully acctylated carbamate and hypotensive thiocarbamate glycosides
from *Moringa oleifera*. *Phytochemistry* 1995;38:p.957-963.
[189]Faizi S, BS Siddiqui, et al. Isolation and structure elucidation of
novel hypotensive agents, niazinin A, niazinin B, niazimicin and
niaziminin A plus B from *Moringa oleifera*: The first naturally
occurring thiocarbamates. *Journal of the Chemical Society Perkin
Transactions*. 1992;I(23):p.3237-3241.
[190] Faizi S, et al. Novel hypotensive agents, niazimin A, niazimin B,
niazicin A and niazicin B from *Moringa oleifera*: Isolation of first
naturally occurring carbamates. *Journal of the Chemical Society
Perkin Transactions I:* 1994;p.3035-3040.
[191] Faizi S, Siddiqui B S, Saleem R, Aftab K, Shaheen F, Gilani A H.
Isolation and structure elucidation of new nitrile and mustard oil
glycosides from *Moringa oleifera* and their effect on blood pressure.
Journal of Natural Products 1994;57:p.1256-1261.
[192] Gilani A H, Aftab K, Suria A, Siddiqui S, Saleem R, Siddiqui B S,
Faizi S. Pharmacological studies on hypotensive and spasmolytic
activities of pure compounds from *Moringa oleifera*. *Phytotherapy
Research* 1994;8(2):p.87-91.

Cardiovascular related disease ranks as the number one killer annually in the United States and the concomitant expenses associated with it have a huge impact globally. With the documented cholesterol and hypertension reduction benefits, the introduction of Moringa based products into a preventive or supplemental regimen may be enough to shift the intensity of the worldwide health effects.

AGE-RELATED MACULAR DEGENERATION & EYE DISEASE

Age related macular degeneration (AMD) is the leading cause of irreversible blindness in developed countries.[194] When considering chronic disease and aging, the fact that cataracts are diagnosed in approximately eighty percent (80%) of the population over the age of seventy five (75),[195] highly qualifies this disorder as a chronic disease of epidemic proportions. The pathophysiology of degenerating eye health seems to involve damage done by exposure to excessive blue light.[196] Lutein and zeaxanthin, carotenoid antioxidants, highly

---

[193] Limaye D A, Nimbkar A Y, Jain R, Ahmad M.(1995) Cardiovascular effects of the aqueous extract of Moringa pterygosperma. Phytotherapy Research 1995;9:p.37-40.
[194] Van Leeuwen R, Boekhoorn S, Vingerling J R, Witteman C M, et al. Dietary intake of antioxidants and risk of age-related macular degeneration. JAMA. 2005; 294:p3101-3107.
[195]Deming D M, Boileau T, Heintz K H, Arkinson C A, Erdman J W Jr. Carotenoids: Linking chemistry, absorption, and metabolism to potential roles in human health and disease. In Cadenas E, and Packer L, (Eds). Handbook of Antioxidants. Marcel-Dekker. New York. 2002; p189-221.
[196] Bone R A, Landrum J T, Guerra L H, Ruiz C A. Lutein and zeaxanthin dietary dietary supplements raise macular pigment density and serum concentrations of these carotenoids in humans. J of Nutr. 2003; 133:p992-998.

concentrated in the macula,[197] have been linked to providing protection from this potential threat.[198] [199] The strong case for the decreased risk of AMD is evidenced by the inverse relationship of decreased lutein and zeaxanthin macular content and the increased incidence of disease.[200] [201] Increasing ingestion of foods high in lutein and other beta carotenoids or supplementing with lutein, beta carotene, vitamin C, vitamin E and zinc increases their density in the macular pigments[202] [203] and significantly decreases the risk of AMD in seniors.[204] [205] The significant levels of zinc, vitamin A, carotenoids, and vitamin C in *Moringa oleifera* offers hope in potentially delaying or

[197] Bone R A, Landrum J T, Friedes L M, Gomez C M, et al. Distribution of lutein and zeaxanthin stereoisomers in the human retina. *Experimental Eye Research*. 1997; 64:p211-218.
[198] Sies H, Stahl W. Non-nutritive bioactive constituents of plants: lycopene, lutein and zeaxanthin. *Intl J for Vitamin and Nutritional Research*. 2003; 73:p95-100.
[199] Krinsky N I, Landrum J T, Bone R A. Biologic mechanisms of the protective role of lutein and zeaxanthin in the eye. *Annual Review of Nutrition*. 2003; 23:p171-201.
[200] Bone R A, Landrum J T, Dixon Z, Chen Y, Liercna C M. Lutein and zeaxanthin in the eyes, serum and dict of human subjects. *Experimental Eye Research*. 2000; 71:p239-245
[201] Bernstein P S, Zhao D Y, Wintch S W, Ermakov I V, et al. Resonance Raman measurement of macular carotenoids in normal subjects and in age-related macular degeneration. *Ophthalmology*. 2002; 109:p1780-1787.
[202] Bone R A, Landrum J T, Guerra L H, Ruiz C A. Lutein and zeaxanthin dietary dietary supplements raise macular pigment density and serum concentrations of these carotenoids in humans. *J of Nutr*. 2003; 133:p992-998.
[203] Mares-Perlman J A, Fisher A I, Klein R, et al. Lutein and zeaxanthin in the diet and serum and their relation to age-related maculopathy in the third National Health and Nutrition Examination Survey. *Am J Epidemiol*. 2001; 153:p424-432
[204] van Leeuwen R, Boekhoorn S, Vingerling J R, Witteman C M, et al. Dietary intake of antioxidants and risk of age-related macular degeneration. *JAMA*. 2005; 294:p3101-3107.
[205] Mares J A. Potential value of antioxidant-rich foods in slowing age-related macular degeneration. *Arch Ophthamol*. 2006; 124(9):p1339-1340.

offsetting AMD. [206] [207] [208] [209] [210] [211] Associate Professor of physical and industrial chemistry, J. T. Barminas and his group (1998) found that Moringa also had extremely high levels of zinc (25.5 mg per100 g).[212] The research truly linking the nutrient abilities of Moringa and AMD are found in the paper of Seddon (1994) where the combination of vitamins A C and E demonstrated benefits for macular degeneration.[213]

ALZHEIMER'S DISEASE (AD)

Alzheimer's Disease   (AD) is a progressive, irreversible brain disorder with no known cause or cure affecting more than six million Americans. The 2009 World Alzheimer's Report estimates 35 million people worldwide are living with Alzheimer's and other forms of dementia. Unfortunately this disease leads to a rapid

[206]Fuglie L J. *The Miracle Tree: Moringa oleifera: Natural Nutrition for the Tropics*. Church World Service, Dakar. 1999;68pp.
[207]Fahey J W. *Moringa oleifera*: a review of the medical evidence for its nutritional, therapeutic, and prophylactic properties. *Trees for Life Journal*. 2005;1(5) p. 1-13.
[208] Geervani P, Devi A. Influence of protein and fat on the utilisation of carotene from drumstick (*Moringa oleifera*) leaves. *Indian J Med Res*. 1981;74:p.548-553.
[209] Delisle H, Bakari S, et al. Provitamin A content of traditional green leaves from Niger. *Cahiers Agricultures* 1997;6(6):p,553-560.
[210] Babu S C. Rural nutrition interventions with indigenous plant foods: a case study of vitamin deficiency in Malawi. International Food Policy Research Institute, Washington, DC. *Biotechnology, Agronomy Soc. Environ*. 2000 ;4(3):p.169-179.
[211] Nambiar V S, Seshadri S. Bioavailability trials of beta-carotene from fresh and dehydrated leaves of *Moringa oleifera* in a rat model. *Plant Foods for Human Nutrition*. 2001;56(1): 83-95.
[212] Barminas J T, Charles M, Emmanuel D. Mineral composition of non-conventional leafy vegetables. *Plant Foods for Human Nutrition* Dordrecht 1998;53(1):p.29-36.
[213] Seddon J M, Ajani U A, Sperduto R D, et al.Dietary carotenoids, vitamins A, C, and E, and advanced age-related macular degeneration. Eye Disease Case-Control Study Group. *JAMA*. 1994; 272(18):p.1413-1420.

functional decline. The clinical cause of Alzheimer's disease is related to amyloid peptide microtubule deposits (tau protein), neurofibril entanglement and inflammation. Neurodegenerative disorders such as Alzheimer's, Parkinson's and dementias are predominantly caused by oxidative damage.[214] The worldwide annual costs for caring for Alzheimer's sufferers was $604 billion, including $96-billion in direct medical care, $255-billion for residential care such as nursing homes, and $253-billion in unpaid labour by family caregivers.[215]

Investigations have shown promising results with the role of antioxidants delaying the onset and progression of Alzheimer's Disease by protecting against cerebral oxidative stress and abnormal protein metabolism.[216] This has been confirmed on autopsy findings that signs of oxidative damage are consistently found in patients with AD and neurodegenerative disorders.[217] Non-steroidal anti-inflammatory benefits of polysaccharides and triterpenoids found in many species of plants may provide the ability to reduce inflammation in the brain reducing the risk for suffering from this disorder.[218] Although the research was conducted using genetically modified drosophila, Dr. D. Dias-Santagata and her fellow researchers believe that antioxidants may be the therapeutic approach to delay or

[214] Mayo J C, Sainz R M, Tan D X, Antolin I, Rodriguez C, Reiter R J. Melatonin and parkinson's disease. *Endocrine*. 2005; 27:p169-178.
[215] http://www.theglobeandmail.com/life/health/dementia/alarming-rise-in-dementia-comes-with-a-crippling-price-tag/article1715781/
[216] Calabrese V, Butterfield D A, Stella A M. Nutritional antioxidants and the heme pathway of stress tolerance: novel targets for neuroprotection in Alzheimer's disease. *Ital J Biochem*. 2003; Dec: (52)4:p177-181.
[217] Dias-Santagata D, Fulga T A, Duttaroy A, Feany M B. Oxidative stress mediates tau-induced neurodegeneration in Drosophila. *J. Clin. Invest*. 2007; 117:p236-245
[218]Fisher H W. Reishi Rescue: R & R for Your Immune System. Wood Publishing. Toronto. 2005; p31.

avoid the onset of AD and other neurodegenerative disorders.[219]

Njoku (1997) found that Moringa demonstrated significant antioxidant and detoxification properties, both relevant in delaying the onset or the prevention of Alzheimer's.[220] A later study, Siddhuraju (2003) corroborated the strong antioxidant activity of the drumstick tree (*Moringa oleifera*).[221]

It has been found recently that the *Moringa oleifera* leaf extract, which is not toxic at higher concentrations, enhances memory and provides substantial antioxidants like vitamin C and E to combat oxidative stress in AD.[222] [223] [224] [225] Many studies substantiate that physiological factors

[219] Dias-Santagata D, Fulga T A, Duttaroy A, Feany M B. Oxidative stress mediates tau-induced neurodegeneration in Drosophila. *J. Clin. Invest.* 2007; 117:p236-245.

[220] Njoku O U, Adikwu M U. Investigation on some physico-chemical antioxidant and toxicological properties of *Moringa oleifera* seed oil. *Acta Pharmaceutica Zagreb*. 1997;47(4):p.87-290.

[221] Siddhuraju P, Becker K. Antioxidant properties of various solvent extracts of total phenolic constituents from three different agroclimatic origins of drumstick tree (*Moringa oleifera* Lam.) leaves. *Journal of Agricultural and Food Chemistry*. 2003;51:p. 2144-2155.

[222] Ganguly R, Hazra R, Ray K, Guha D. Effect of Moringa oleifera in experimental model of Alzheimer's disease: Role of antioxidants. *Ann Neurosci*. 2005;12:p.36-9.

[223] Mohan M, Kaul N, Punekar A, Girnar R, Junnare P, Patil L. Nootropic activity of Moringa oleifera leaves. *J Nat Remedies*. 2005;5:p.59-62.

[224] Majumdar K, Gupta M, Chakrobarty S, Pal DK. Evaluation of hematological and hepatorenal functions of methanolic extract of Moringa oleifera Lam. root treated mice. *Indian J Exp Biol*. 1999;37:p.612-614.

[225] Ganguly R, Guha D. Protective role of an Indian herb, Moringa oleifera in memory impairment by high altitude hypoxic exposure: Possible role of monoamines. *Biogenic Amines*. 2006;20:p.121-33.

involved in the memory loss are affected by *Moringa oleifera* extracts.[226]

DIABETES

North America is being ravaged by both obesity and diabetes which go hand in hand. There are two types of diabetes, which is a disease affecting the levels of serum glucose. Both types can be affected by diet. In type I diabetes the pancreas can no longer produce insulin and exogenous insulin that is needed to control serum glucose levels. With type II diabetes, the body no longer responds to the insulin secreted by the pancreas and thus serum glucose levels run out of control. Approximately 26 million Americans have diabetes, according to 2011 estimates from the Centers for Disease Control and Prevention (CDC); 8.3% of the total population. Furthermore, an estimated 79 million U.S. adults have prediabetes, a condition in which blood sugar levels are higher than normal, but not high enough to be diagnosed as diabetes.[227] As a result of these large numbers, much research has been done in the relationship between diet, nutrition and diabetes.[228] Diabetes is the major cause of heart disease and stroke and the seventh leading cause of death in the United States and costs America $174 billion annually.[229]

The Moringa tree has been shown to supply benefits to combat this globally pervasive disease through a number

---

[226] Obulesu O, Rao D M. Effect of plant extracts on Alzheimer's disease: An insight into therapeutic avenues. *J Neurosciences in Rural Practice*. 2011;2(1):p.56-61.
[227] CDC Publications and Products: National Diabetes Fact Sheet. <http://www.cdc.gov/diabetes/pubs/estimates05.htm#prev.
[228] Franz M J, Bantle J P, Beebe R D, Brunzell J D, et al. Evidence-based nutrition principles and recommendations for the treatment and prevention of diabetes and related complications. *Diabetes Care*. 2002; 25:p148-198.
[229] http://www.cdc.gov/diabetes/pubs/pdf/ndfs_2011.pdf

of mechanisms that lead to the decrease of serum glucose.[230][231][232][233][234]

The dialogue from various researchers indicates that trace minerals such as potassium, magnesium, chromium and zinc deficiencies may have an effect on carbohydrate intolerance.[235][236][237] Zinc has catalytic functions involving insulin degradation, hundreds of enzymes, thousands of proteins and the ability to regulate many physiological functions.[238] Jansen et al (2009) found that zinc, can aid in normalizing the negative effects of diabetes mellitus by improving glycemic control in type I and type II diabetes.[239] Many of the enzyme systems which utilize zinc are involved with the metabolism of blood sugar, and make

---

[230]Asres K. The major constituents of the acetone fraction of Ethiopian *Moringa stenopetala* leaves. *Mansoura Journal of Pharmacological Science*. 1995;11(1):p.55-64.

[231] Faizi S, Siddiqui B S, Saleem R, Aftab K, Shaheen F, Gilani A H. Bioactive Compounds from the leaves and pods of *Moringa oleifera*. *New Trends in Natural Products Chemistry* 1998;p.175-183.

[232] Kar A, Choundhary B, Bandyopadhyay N. Preliminary studies on the inorganic constituents of some indigenous hypoglycaemic herbs on oral glucose tolerance test. *J Ethnopharmacology*. 1999;64(2):p.179-184.

[233] Kar A, Choundhary B, Bandyopadhyay N. Comparative evaluation of hypoglycaemic activity of some Indian medicinal plants in alloxan diabetic rats. *J Ethnopharmacol*. 2003;Jan; 84 (1):p.105-108.

[234] Makonnen E, Hunde A, Damecha G. Hypoglycaemic effect of *Moringa stenopetala* aqueous extract in rabbits. *Phytotherapy Research* 1997;11:p.147-148

[235]Franz M J, Bantle J P, Beebe R D, Brunzell J D, et al. Evidence-based nutrition principles and recommendations for the treatment and prevention of diabetes and related complications. *Diabetes Care*.

[236] Mooradian A D, Failla M, Hoogwerf B, Maryniuk M, et al. Selected vitamins and minerals in diabetes. *Diabetes Care*. 1994; 17:p464–479.

[237] Mooradian AD: Micronutrients in diabetes mellitus. In *Drugs, Diet and Disease2*. 1999; p183–200.

[238] Maret W. Zinc and Diabetes. *Biometals*. 2005;18(4):p.293-294.

[239] Jansen J, Karges W, Rink L. Zinc and diabetes - clinical links and molecular mechanisms. *J Nut Biochem*. 2009;20(6):p.399-417.

zinc a natural catalyst for insulin secretion.[240] Moringa leaves provide a significant amount of zinc.[241] [242]

Chromium has been linked to decreasing serum glucose, glucose intolerance, and other aspects of relieving the symptoms of diabetes.[243] [244] [245] [246] The moringaceae family provides the anti-inflammatory trace mineral, chromium.[247] [248] Overall, the investigations for vitamin and mineral benefits for diabetes have yielded mixed results, and have only shown true benefit when distinctive nutrient deficiencies were present, but judging from the average sugar and carbohydrate laden western diet, these deficiencies abound .

[240] Jansen J, Karges W, Rink L. Zinc and diabetes - clinical links and molecular mechanisms. *J Nut Biochem*. 2009;20(6):p.399-417.

[241] Barminas J T, Charles M, Emmanuel D. Mineral composition of non-conventional leafy vegetables. *Plant Foods for Human Nutrition* Dordrecht 1998;53(1):p.29-36.

[242] Fuglie L J. *The Miracle Tree: Moringa oleifera: Natural Nutrition for the Tropics*. Church World Service, Dakar. 1999;68 pp.

[243] Anderson R A, Cheng N, Bryden N A, Polansky M M, et al. Beneficial effects of chromium for people with diabetes. *Diabetes*. 1997; 46:p1786–1791.

[244] Cheng N, Zhu X, Shi H, Wu W, Chi J, et al. Follow-up survey of people in China with type 2 diabetes mellitus consuming supplemental chromium. *J Trace Elem Exp Med*. 1999; (12):p55–60.

[245] Ravina A, Slezak L, Rubal A, Mirsky N. Clinical use of trace element chromium (III) in the treatment of diabetes mellitus. *J Trace Elem Exp Med*. 1995; 8:p183–190.

[246] Cefalu WT, Bell-Farrow AD, Stegner J, Wang ZQ, King T, Morgan, Terry JG: Effect of chromium picolinate on insulin sensitivity in vivo. *J Trace Elem Exp Med*. 1999; (12):p71–83.

[247] Ndiaye M, Dieye A M, Mariko F, Tall A, Sall Diallo A, Faye B. Contribution to the study of the anti-inflammatory activity of Moringa oleifera (moringaceae). *Dakar Med*, 2002;47(2):p.210-212.

[248] Fuglie L J. *The Miracle Tree: Moringa oleifera: Natural Nutrition for the Tropics*. Church World Service, Dakar. 1999;68 pp.

OSTEOPOROSIS

Osteoporosis is a disease characterized by low bone mass and micro-architectural deterioration of bone tissue,[249] and affects more than twenty-eight million (28,000,000) people in the United States alone.[250] Hundreds of thousands of hip and femoral fractures occur annually and twenty-five percent (25%) of these individuals die within a year.[251] Although there are many factors affecting this disease (malabsorption syndromes etc), the focal point of the process of calcium absorption is the dietary presence of the nutrients, calcium, magnesium, and vitamin D.[252] [253] The dietary needs of osteoporosis are completely fulfilled by the nutrition available from *Moringa oleifera*. This plant that can grow virtually with no water, provides calcium and magnesium and in more than ample quantities.[254] [255] [256] [257] One ounce of Moringa leaf provides

---

[249] Brunader R, Shelton D K. Radiologic Bone Assessment in the Evaluation of Osteoporosis. *Am Fam Physician*. 2002; p1357-1364.

[250] NIH Consensus Statement. Osteoporosis Prevention, Diagnosis, and Therapy. 2000; 17(1):p1-36.

[251] Langton C M. Ultrasound Measurement of Cancellous Bone for the Assessment of osteoporosis.
<http://www.hull.ac.uk/medphys/QUS1.doc.

[252] Bronner F. Calcium Absorption: A paradigm for mineral absorption. *J Nutr*. 1998; 128:p917-920

[253] NIH Consensus Development Panel on Osteoporosis Prevention, Diagnosis, and Therapy. Osteoporosis Prevention Diagnosis, and Therapy. *JAMA*. 2001; 285:p785-795.

[254] Babu S C. Rural nutrition interventions with indigenous plant foods: a case study of vitamin deficiency in Malawi. International Food Policy Research Institute, Washington, DC. *Biotechnology, Agronomy Soc. Environ*. 2000 ;4(3):p.169-179.

[255] Fuglie L J. *The Miracle Tree: Moringa oleifera: Natural Nutrition for the Tropics*. Church World Service, Dakar. 1999;68 pp.

[256] Fahey J W. *Moringa oleifera*: a review of the medical evidence for its nutritional, therapeutic, and prophylactic properties. *Trees for Life Journal*. 2005;1(5) p. 1-13.

[257] Pankaja N, Prakash J.(1994) Availability of calcium from kilkeerai (*Amaranthus tricolor*) and drumstick (*Moringa oleifera*) greens in weanling rats. *Nahrung* 1994;38:p.199-203.

more than the recommended daily allowance (RDA) of calcium (125%) and 61% of the magnesium.[258]

The maintenance of the integrity of all of the physiological parameters necessary to ensure good health can be found in what we eat. As Hippocrates said two thousand years ago, "Let food be your medicine and medicine be your food." This is an adage that we can abide by. Poor nutrition has been linked to the major chronic diseases, immune system dysfunction and premature aging that are affecting the global population to a decreased quality of life. Table X below shows the actual quantities of life-sustaining nutrition contained in *Moringa oleifera*.

The current position based on the investigative findings demonstrates a suggested connection between nutritional deficiencies, chronic disease, and aging. There is now more than marginal corroboration, and new objective measurement techniques to be used in future studies will confirm this beyond the shadow of a doubt.

The case to support nutrient supplementation is strong, based on the fact that nutrients, such as folate, and antioxidants, (carotenoids and vitamins C and E), when ingested as distinct compounds are extremely bioavailable, often more than most whole foods.[259] [260] "If used consistently, supplements can ensure adequate intakes of specific nutrients in targeted groups."[261]

---

[258] Price M L. *The Moringa Tree*. ECHO Technical Note. Educational Concerns for Hunger Organization. N. Ft. Meyers, FL. 1985.
[259] Hannon-Fletcher M P, Armstrong N C, Scott J M, et al. Determining bioavailability of food folates in a controlled interventions study. *Am J Clin Nutr*. 2004; 80:p911-918.
[260] Brown E D, Micozzi M S, Craft M E, et al. Plasma carotenoids in normal men after a single ingestion of vegetables or purified beta-carotene. *Am J Clin Nutr*. 1989; 49:p1258-1265.
[261] Lichtenstein A H, Russell R M. Essential Nutrients: Food or Supplements? Where Should the Emphasis Be? *JAMA*. 2005; 294:p351-358.

TABLE II
Nutrient Content *Moringa oleifera* Per 100 grams[262]

Category	Pods	Leaves	Leaf Powder
Calories	26	92	205
Protein (g)	2.5	6.7	27.1
Fat (g)	0.1	1.7	2.3
Carbohydrate (g)	3.7	13.4	38.2
Fiber (g)	4.8	0.9	19.2
Minerals (g)	2.0	2.3	-
Calcium (mg)	30	440	2003
Magnesium (mg)	24	24	368
Phosphorus (mg)	110	70	204
Potassium (mg)	259	259	1324
Copper (mg)	3.1	1.1	0.7
Iron (mg)	5.3	7	28.2
Sulphur (mg)	137	137	870
Oxalic Acid (mg)	10	101	1.6%
Vitamin A (beta carotene) (mg)	0.11	6.8	16.3
Vitamin B choline (mg)	423	423	8.2
Vitamin B1 thiamine (mg)	0.5	0.21	2.64
Vitamin B2 riboflavin (mg)	0.7	0.5	20,5
Vitmin B3 (mg)	0.2	0.8	8.2
Vitamin C(Ascorbic Acid) (mg)	120	220	17.3
Vitamin E (tocopherol acetate) (mg)	-	-	113

From an epidemiological perspective, the relationships between nutrition and disease have been identified. *Moringa oleifera* certainly holds an esteemed

---

[262] Fuglie L J. *The Miracle Tree: Moringa oleifera: Natural Nutrition for the Tropics*. Church World Service, Dakar. 1999;68 pp.

position as a source of phytonutrients with the ability to affect human health. [263] [264] [265]

It might be easy enough to suggest that everyone eat five to ten servings of fruit and vegetables daily or a commensurate amount of nutritional supplementation, but three decades of treating patients has shown that there are inherent difficulties with individual compliance to this regimen. Introduction of, what may be considered by some to be the 'drumstick' panacea, will make this process much easier. The demographics will demonstrate significant decreases to the incidence of the previously discussed diseases and perhaps the morbidity and dysfunction associated with the aging process and nutritional maladies will be decreased through the proper use of foods such as *Moringa oleifera* heralded in folk literature to cure more than three hundred diseases. [266] [267]

---

[263] Fuglie L J. *The Miracle Tree: Moringa oleifera: Natural Nutrition for the Tropics*. Church World Service, Dakar. 1999;68 pp.
[264] Fahey J W. *Moringa oleifera*: a review of the medical evidence for its nutritional, therapeutic, and prophylactic properties. *Trees for Life Journal*. 2005;1(5) p. 1-13.
[265] Babu S C. Rural nutrition interventions with indigenous plant foods: a case study of vitamin deficiency in Malawi. International Food Policy Research Institute, Washington, DC. *Biotechnology, Agronomy Soc. Environ*. 2000 ;4(3):p.169-179.
[266] Fuglie L J. *The Miracle Tree: Moringa oleifera: Natural Nutrition for the Tropics*. Church World Service, Dakar. 1999;68 pp.
[267] Fahey J W. *Moringa oleifera*: a review of the medical evidence for its nutritional, therapeutic, and prophylactic properties. *Trees for Life Journal*. 2005;1(5) p. 1-13.

CHAPTER 4

OVERCOMING DISEASE: DEFENDING IMMUNE SYSTEM ASSAULT

"If we could give every individual the right amount of nourishment and exercise, not too little and not too much, we would have found the safest way to health."

Hippocrates

Why do we not have perfect health always? What separates us from everything else on the planet? What establishes individuals as distinct and separate entities? What is our sole protection against the environment? The answer is our immune system. Our initial lines of defense are the membranes (skin and mucous membranes) that separate us from the environment.[268] We have two square metres of skin and over four hundred square metres of mucous membrane.

In the hostile environment in which we reside, we need protection from the multitude of microorganisms and toxins that are omnipresent. We can't see these invaders and probably will not notice them until we are adversely affected, but that doesn't lessen the impact they can have on us. Dr. Yulius Poplyansky, Director of the International

---

[268] Toyokawa H, Yoichi Matsui, et al. Promotive Effects of Far-Infrared Ray on Full-Thickness Skin Wound Healing in Rats. Experimental Biology and Medicine. 2003; 228: p724-729.

Foundation for Innovative Medicine, states, "Every severe and chronic disease is directly associated with immune dysfunction".[269] To corroborate this, research has shown that decreased NK (Natural Killer) cell activity levels are present with almost all illnesses.[270] Dr. Jesse Stoff, M.D., nationally known author, lecturer and clinical researcher, suggests that with an intact immune system there can be no chronic or severe disease.[271] Copious toxicity will have deleterious effects on our immune system. In the previous chapter we saw how Moringa can beneficially affect natural killer cells.

Reduced to simplest terms, the immune system has two functions: identify self from non-self and to destroy, eliminate, or store non-self and any form of toxin present in the body that acts as a stressor to the immune system. This can only work when the immune system and all of the components function optimally. Complications arise from miscommunication when the body incorrectly identifies an invader and/or attacks 'self' (auto-immune diseases such as ankylosing spondylitis, diabetes, multiple sclerosis, fibromyalgia, chronic fatigue syndrome, psoriasis, rheumatoid arthritis, ulcerative colitis, vitiligo, systemic lupus and approximately seventy-five more)[272] or the immune system fails to identify an invader (or wrongly manufactured cell such as cancer).[273] Or the immune

---

[269] Immune Solutions In Practice. Immune Dysfunction and Modulation. 2002.
<http://www.immunesolutions.net/clinical_studies.php.
[270] Stoff J. An Examination of Immune Response Modulation in Humans by Antigen Infused Dialyzable Bovine Colostrum/Whey Extract Using A Double Blind Study. Tucson. Immune Consultants. 2001 p1.
[271] Stoff J. Toronto Lecture. December 7, 2002.
[272] Lane William, Baxter Susan. Immune Power. Garden City Park, New York. Avery Publishing Group. 1999; p12-13, 81-85.
[273] Simone C. Cancer & Nutrition. Garden City Park, New York. Avery Publishing Group. 1992; p45.

system is compromised due to poor nutrition[274], infection, trauma, toxicity or stress to the extent that it is unable to overcome the immune insult.[275]

Autoimmune disorders, such as any of the rheumatoid arthritises, are a pure example of disease where the body attacks itself.[276] All these errors result in some form of disease. There are several areas that can stress the immune system and most of these can be affected beneficially to varying degrees by our actions.

Every biological contaminant, virus, bacteria, pollen, mold, mildew, spore, dander, and dust mite that is airborne has the ability to enter your body and cause your immune system to react. The pathway is clear. Access may be granted through your mouth, nose, eyes, ears or any external opening. Biological contaminants are not the only invaders with which one has to be concerned.

We may not be aware of the massive amount of immune system insults we face daily and we will not be, unless something goes wrong. This may very well be the reason that there is so much sickness and disease running rampant through our society.

Many of us believe that headache, fatigue, aches, pains, allergies, digestive difficulties, mucus build-up and chemical sensitivity that affect a large percentage of the population are due to unknown causes or environmental factors. Epstein (2003) suggests that our lack of awareness

---

[274] Simone C. Cancer & Nutrition. Garden City Park, New York. Avery Publishing Group. 1992; p43
[275] Stoff J. An Examination of Immune Response Modulation in Humans by Antigen Infused Dialyzable Bovine Colostrum/Whey Extract Using A Double Blind Study. Tucson. Immune Consultants. January 2001.
[276] Berkow R, Talbott J, Eds. The Merck Manual Thirteenth Edition. Rahway. Merck Sharpe and Dohme Research Laboratories. 1977; p 241-243.

is due, in part, to the fact that the major focus of many influential groups has not made us aware of the potential problem areas. For example "the cancer establishment's mindset remains fixated on 'secondary' prevention or damage control-- screening, diagnosis and chemoprevention (the use of drugs or nutrients to reduce risks from prior avoidable carcinogenic exposures)—and treatment."[277]   This statement is indicative of the fact that there are precautions and preventive actions that every individual can take to minimize the chances of reducing the quality of their health. Big business will not protect us from themselves. They have a different agenda.

We can only react to threats to our health when we know that they indeed are threats. "The U.S. cancer establishment conducts minimal research on avoidable exposures to a wide range of industrial carcinogens contaminating the totality of the environment—air, water, soil, the workplace, and consumer products—carcinogenic prescription drugs and low dose diagnostic medical radiation."[278]   Electromagnetic radiation, which is now totally pervasive in our environment, is another insult challenging our immune system and our health and once again, no one is stepping up with the real information.

There is no one to blame, but we need all of the help we can get. This philosophy is consistent with North American allopathic therapeutics: find out what is causing the disease and kill it pharmaceutically before the host dies. Do not take into consideration the toxic effects of the pharmaceuticals being put into our systems.

What are the signs of a weakened immune system? Is it possible that we are so affected that we have come to

[277] Epstein S. The Stop Cancer Before It Starts Campaign. Chicago. The Cancer Prevention Coalition. February 2003; p4.
[278] Epstein S. The Stop Cancer Before It Starts Campaign. Chicago. The Cancer Prevention Coalition. February 2003;p4

accept it as normal? Recurring infections, chronic tiredness, slower healing, allergies, inflammation and colds or flu several times a year are not just 'bad luck'. Your immune system has been affected, and now it is time to adopt a different approach.

There is another philosophy and that is to take a preventive approach. You will see how Moringa fits into this equation. According to Fahey (2005), "Moringa appears to be a nutritional and medical cornucopia."[279] Since we only have a finite amount of energy and immune capability, there are a number of protocols one might adopt to avoid toxicity. This preventive approach can improve your health and in doing so allow your body to better combat all types of disease.

INFECTIOUS AGENTS

Our environment is rife with infectious agents.[280] They are not visible to the naked eye but the fact that we cannot see them does not make them go away. Disease runs rampant because our immune systems are constantly under attack.[281] In the late eighteenth century, the early surgeons performed masterful work yet the patients often died from the subsequent bacterial infections. It was not until Louis Pasteur's acute observations in the late 1860's that the world was made aware of the presence of bacteria on most surfaces.[282] Pathogenic microorganisms are everywhere and it is only our immune system that keeps us healthy.

---

[279] Fahey J W. *Moringa oleifera*: a review of the medical evidence for its nutritional, therapeutic, and prophylactic properties. *Trees for Life Journal*. 2005;1(5) p. 1-13.
[280] Lane William, Baxter Susan. Immune Power. Garden City Park, New York. Avery Publishing Group. 1999; p43.
[281] Stoff J. The Ultimate Nutrient. Tucson. Insight Consulting Services. 2000; p12.
[282] Lane William, Baxter Susan. Immune Power. Garden City Park, New York. Avery Publishing Group. 1999; p46.

There are at least four thousand viruses that have been named and billions of bacteria.[283] Antibiotics have become less effective and have caused the mutation of antibiotic resistant forms of bacteria.[284] Infectious disease is a direct attack on your immune system. According to Dr. Jesse Stoff, M.D., "Even if you are perfectly healthy, thousands of viruses may be present in your blood, only seventy-five percent (75%) of which have been identified."

Ninety-five percent (95%) of the American population carries the Epstein-Barr virus.[285] This virus has been linked to Chronic Fatigue Syndrome, Fibro-myalgia, and mononucleosis. In 1956 this virus was discovered to be oncogenic or cancer causing and has direct links to breast, prostate and nasopharyngeal cancers as well as leukemias and lymphomas.[286] [287] Murakami et al (1998) found that a phytochemical in the leaves of the Moringa inhibited Epstein-Barr virus growth.[288]

According to the National Center for Infectious Diseases, "cytomegalovirus (CMV) infects between 50% and 85% of adults in the United States by the age of 40."[289]

---

[283] Nature Works. Immune Disorders. 2002.
<http://immunedisorders.homestead.com/booklet/html.
[284] Lane William, Baxter Susan. Immune Power. Garden City Park, New York. Avery Publishing Group. 1999; p50.
[285] Centers for Disease Control and Prevention. Epstein-Barr Virus and infectious Mononucleosis. National Center for Infectious Diseases. October 26, 2002 (updated).
<http://www.cdc.gov/ncidod/diseases/ebv.htm.
[286] Stoff J. Toronto Lecture. December 7, 2002.
[287] Simone C. Cancer & Nutrition. Garden City Park, New York. Avery Publishing Group. 1992; p48.
[288] Murakami A, Kitazono Y, Jiwajinda S, Koshimizu K, Ohigashi H. Niaziminin, a thiocarbamate from the leaves of *Moringa oleifera*, holds a strict structural requirement for inhibition of tumor-promoter-induced Epstein-Barr virus activation. *Planta Medica* 1998;64: p.319-323.
[289] Centers for Disease Control and Prevention. Cytomegalovirus. National Center for Infectious Diseases. October 26, 2002 (updated). <http://www.cdc.gov/ncidod/diseases/cmv.htm

Furthermore "CMV infection is more widespread in developing countries and in areas of lower socioeconomic conditions." Aside from causing pneumonia, retinitis and gastrointestinal disease, cytomegalovirus has been linked to breast and prostate cancer.[290] Sixteen percent (16%) of the population carries the herpes virus. The relevant point here is the importance of the immune system. As long as our immune systems remain relatively intact, these viruses can be held in check, however when the immune system stressors escalate to an overload status, the immune system can make communication errors or be defeated by a more powerful invader.

LYME DISEASE

Lyme disease, also known as borreliosis, is an often times persistent infectious disease most likely caused by at least three species of bacteria belonging to the genus Borrelia . Of these bacteria, Borrelia burgdorferi sensu lato is the main cause of Lyme disease in North America and Borrelia afzelii and garinii cause most European cases. The disease was determined to be one that was a tick-borne disease, however many other sources now suspect a number of other vectors. The true incidence of this disease is difficult to estimate due to a lack of standardized testing protocols, but experts indicate that there are approximately 300,000 cases in the US today and according to the CDC, this number may be ten times greater. Intermittently, symptoms such as arthritic inflammatory conditions persist after the infection has been eliminated by antibiotics. This fact leads to the likelihood that Borrelia may cause an autoimmune response, and furthermore it may be considered to be a pathogen induced autoimmune disease[291]

---

[290] ibid.
[291] Singh S K, Girshik H J. Lyme borreliosis: from infection to autoimmunity. *Clin Microbiol Infect*. 2004;10(7):p.598-614.

Early symptoms may include fever, headache,
fatigue, depression, and a characteristic circular skin rash
called erythema migrans (looks like a target) but the extent
of symptoms may extend to a diversity involving the joints,
heart, and CNS (central nervous system).[292] Lyme disease
has commonly been misdiagnosed as multiple sclerosis
(MS), rheumatoid arthritis, fibromyalgia, chronic fatigue
syndrome (CFS), lupus, or other autoimmune and
neurodegenerative diseases and has often been called the
"great imitator"[293] [294] [295] [296] [297] The significance of
mentioning Lyme Disease in a book about Moringa, quite
frankly, is due to the fact that *Moringa oleifera* is an antipyretic,[298] [299] [300] anti-inflammatory,[301] [302] and possesses a

---

[292] Cairns V, Godwin J. Post-Lyme borreliosis syndrome: a meta-
analysis of reported symptoms. *Int J Epidemiol*. 2005;34(6):p.1340-
1345.
[293] Pachner A R. Neurologic manifestations of Lyme disease, the new
"great imitator". *Rev Infect Dis*. 1989;11 Suppl 6:pS1482-1486.
[294] Burch J B, Reif J S, Pittrat C A, Keefe T J, Yost M G. Cellular
telephone use and excretion of a urinary melatonin metabolite. In:
Annual review of Research in Biological Effects of electric and
magnetic fields from the generation, delivery and use of electricity. San
Diego. 1997; Nov. 9-13: p.52.
[295] Reiter R J, Tan D X, Pappolla M A. Melatonin relieves the neural
oxidative burden that contributes to dementias. *Ann N Y Acad Sci*.
2004; 1035:p179-196.
[296] Havas M, Stetzer D. Graham/Stetzer Filters Improve Power Quality
in Homes and Schools and Reduce Blood Sugar Levels in Diabetics,
Multiple Sclerosis Symptoms, and Headaches. International Scientific
Conference on Childhood Leukemia. 6th-10th September, London.
2004.
[297] Freiburger Appeal. Umwelt.medizin.gesellschaft. 2003;p.35-36.
http://www.igumed.de/images/fa_1_03.pdf
[298] Hukkeri V I, Nagathan C V, Karadi R V, Patil B S. Antipyretic and
wound healing activities of Moringa oleifera Lam. In rats. *Indian J
Pharmaceutical Sciences*. 2006;68(1):p.124-126
[299]Holst S. *Moringa: Nature's Medicine Cabinet*. Sierra Sunrise
Publishing, Sherman Oaks, CA. 2000.128 pp.
[300] Singh K K, Kumar K. Ethnotherapeutics of some medicinal plants
used as antipyretic agents among the tribals of India. *Journal of
Economic and Taxonomic Botany*. 1999;23(1): p.135-141.

broad spectrum of antibiotic capabilities.[303] [304] [305] A
Moringa dietary protocol makes perfect sense to combat the
ravages of Lyme disease. Renowned Moringa researcher,
Lowell Fuglie, in his book, The Miracle Tree, outlines the
ability of Moringa to reduce swelling, reduce joint pain,
arthritic pain, and a host of anti-bacterial, antibiotic
functions that would vault this miracle tree into the
category of a virtual panacea, especially where Lyme
disease is concerned.

Every time you ingest, inhale or absorb any toxin
your immune system must deal with it. Dr. Bert Berkson,
consultant to the National Centers for Disease Control and
Prevention and Professor of Applied Biology at New
Mexico State states, "your immune system is constantly
laboring to remove toxins from your bloodstream and
tissues. These pollutants may be city smog, industrial
chemicals, herbicides or pesticides. If you smoke you are
exposing yourself to additional poisons. If you are a heavy

---

[301] Caceres A, Saravia A, Rizzo S, Zabala L, Leon E D, Nave F.
Pharmacological properties of Moringa oleifera. 2: Screening for
antispasmodic, anti-inflammatory and diuretic activity. J
Ethnopharmacol 1992;36:p.233-7.
[302] Ezeamuzie I C, Ambakederemo A W, et al. Antiinflammatory
effects of Moringa oleifera root extract. Int J Pharmacognosy.
1996;34(3):p.207-212.
[303] Das B R, Kurup P A, Narasimha Rao P L, Ramaswamy A S.
Antibiotic principle from Moringa pterygosperma. Part VIII. Some
pharma-cological properties and in vivo action of pterygospermin and
related compounds. Indian J Med Res. 1957;45:p.197-206.
[304] Bennett R N, Mellon F A, Foidl N, Pratt J H, DuPont M S, Perkins
L, Kroon P A. Profiling glucosinolates and phenolics in vegetative and
reproductive tissues of the multi-purpose trees Moringa oleifera L.
(Horseradish tree) and Moringa stenopetala L. J Agricultural and Food
Chemistry. 2003;51: p.3546-3553.
[305] Fahey J W, Zalcmann A T, Talalay P. The chemical diversity and
distribution of glucosinolates and isothiocyanates among plants.
Phytochemistry. 2001;56(1):p.5-51.

alcohol user, the same is true."[306] When you compound this with the ambient pathogenic presence in our environment, without taking proper steps, we are heading for an immune system crash.

The signs and symptoms of this immune system crash encompass a diverse range. Pains such as headache, backache, joint pain, and chest pain (angina pectoris) are only the tip of the iceberg. This crash may express itself through: coughing, colds, sinus problems, wheezing, sore throat, runny nose, sneezing, fever, neck stiffness, circulatory deficits, increased serum cholesterol or triglycerides, sleeping problems, fatigue, itchy eyes or nose, dizziness, immune weakness, sensitivity to environmental stimuli, anxiety, depression, mood swings, fatigue, rashes and hives, constipation, indigestion, anorexia, rashes, and bad breath.[307] [308] From the diversity of the disorders it is apparent that immune system function can affect virtually all organ systems and even life itself.

A number of these biological contaminants are pandemic; they will exist anywhere a proper growth media exists. Once again these foreign elements enter the chemical stew and your immune system wants to eliminate them, but it cannot due to a variety of reasons (insufficient water intake, deficient chlorophyll intake, environmental overload etc.) potentially causing health problems. [309] [310]

---

[306] Nature Works. Body Detoxification, Toxins and the Immune System. 2002.
<http://immunedisorders.homestead.com/Detoxification.html
[307] Haas, Elson M. Staying Healthy With Nutrition: The Complete Guide to Diet and Nutritional Medicine. Berkeley, California. Celestial Arts. 1992. p907.
[308] Fletcher D J. Warming up to Far-Infrared. Alternative Medicine Magazine. Jan 2001: 39.
[309] Stoff J. A Study of the Effects of Oral Dietary Supplementation of Antigen Infused Colostrum/Whey Extract Upon Natural Killer Cell Activity in a Healthy Human Population. Scottsdale. Quantum Research Inc. 2001; p2.

Dr. Elson M. Haas explains that, "there are many symptoms of toxicity but the most common signs are headache, fatigue, mucus problems, aches and pains, digestive problems, allergy symptoms and sensitivity to environmental agents like chemicals or perfumes."[311]

When seeking a solution to these problems, the more we can support the immune system through our diets, the less work our immune systems have to do. When we examine Moringa's credentials as an anti-bacterial, anti-viral and anti-fungal, it is easy to understand why there will be less work for our immune system to do.

Researchers such as Das and Kurup (1954, 1957),[312] Rao, Bennett (2003) and Fahey (2001) have shown that Moringa leaf juice contains pterygospermin which breaks down into benzyl isothiocyanate, which is particularly effective against the Pseudomonas aeruginosa bacterium and many other pathogenic microorganisms.[313] [314] [315] Pseudomonas can cause diseases in both animals and humans by infecting people with exposed tissues or a weakened immune system, initiating an inflammatory response. In severe cases, the bacteria can take hold in the

[310] Hueser G. Diagnostic markers in clinical immunotoxicology and neurotoxicology. J Occup Med Toxicol. 1992; 1:p5-9.
[311] Haas, Elson M. Staying Healthy With Nutrition. Berkeley. Celestial Arts. 1992; p905-907.
[312] Das B R, Kurup P A, Narasimha Rao P L. Antibiotic principle from *Moringa pterygosperma*. *Naturwissenschaften* 1954;41:p.66.
[313] Das B R, Kurup P A, Narasimha Rao P L, Ramaswamy A S. Antibiotic principle from *Moringa pterygosperma*. Part VIII. Some pharma-cological properties and in vivo action of pterygospermin and related compounds. *Indian J Med Res*. 1957;45:p.197-206.
[314] Bennett R N, Mellon F A, Foidl N, Pratt J H, DuPont M S, Perkins L, Kroon P A. Profiling glucosinolates and phenolics in vegetative and reproductive tissues of the multi-purpose trees *Moringa oleifera* L. (Horseradish tree) and *Moringa stenopetala* L. *J Agricultural and Food Chemistry*. 2003;51: p.3546-3553.
[315] Fahey J W, Zalcmann A T, Talalay P. The chemical diversity and distribution of glucosinolates and isothiocyanates among plants. *Phytochemistry*. 2001;56(1):p.5-51.

major organs such as the lungs, kidneys, or the urinary
tract, with potentially fatal consequences.

Pseudomonas is not the only bacteria with lethal
consequence. In May 1980, an E. coli outbreak in the
water supply in Walkerton, Ontario, Canada killed seven
people and made about 3,000 people ill. *Moringo oleifera*
not only inhibits E. coli growth but can be used to purify
water as well.[316 317 318 319 320]

Benzyl isothiocyanate has been shown to be
effective in controlling a broad spectrum of bacteria and
fungi.[321 322] Another of the isothiocyanates from Moringa
have been found to be effective against H. pylori.[323 324 325]

---

[316] Viera GH F, Mourão J A, Ângelo Â C, Costa R A, Viera R H.
Antibacterial effect (in vitro) of Moringa oleifera and Annona muricata
against Gram positive and Gram negative bacteria. *Rev Inst Med trop S
Paulo*. 2010;May/June:
[317] Jahn S A, Musnad H A, Burgstaller H., Tree that purifies water:
Cultivating multipurpose Moringaceae in the Sudan. *Unasylva*
1986;38(152):p.23-28.
[318] Berger M R, Habs M, Jahn S A, Schmahl S. Toxicological
assessment of seeds from *Moringa oleifera* and *Moringa stenopetala*,
two highly efficient primary coagulants for domestic water treatment of
tropical raw waters. *East African Medical Journal* 1984;61:p.712-716.
[319] Gassenschmidt U, Jany K D, Tauscher B, Niebergall H. Isolation
and characterization of a flocculating protein from *Moringa oleifera*
Lam. *Biochimica Biophysica Acta*. 1995;1243:p.477-481.
[320] Kumar S, Gopal K (1999) Screening of plant species for inhibition
of bacterial population of raw water. *J Environ Sci & Health: Part A
Toxic Hazardous Substances and Environmental Engineering*.
1994;34(4):p.975-987.
[321] Kjaer A, Malver O, El-Menshawi B, Reisch J. Isothiocyanates in
myrosinase-treated seed extracts of *Moringa peregrina*. *Phytochemistry*
1979;18:p.1485-1487.
[322] Kurup P A, Narasimha Rao P L. Antibiotic principle from *Moringa
pterygosperma*. Part IV. The effect of addition of vitamins and amino
acids on the anti-bacterial activity of pterygospermin. *Indian J Med Res*
1954;42:p.101-107.
[323] Galan M V, Kishan A A, Silverman A A. Oral broccoli sprouts for
the treatment of Helicobacter pylori infection: A preliminary report.
Dig Dis Sci;2004;49(7-8):p.1088-1090.

Helicobacter pylori is a bacteria that is responsible for infecting more than three billion people worldwide. Although about 80% of those infected with H. pylori are symptomless, many suffer from gastritis and ulcers which are characterized by a loss of appetite, nausea, a bloated sensation, burping, vomiting and abdominal pain.[326]

   Much research has been conducted into the antibiotic effects of *Moringa oleifera,* (there are antiviral and antifungal effects as well), and we have just touched upon that. By allowing the active phytonutrients to reduce the workload of the immune system, one would expend less energy and have more energy and components of the immune system available for other functions. In the following table, you will see some of the documented evidence of how diverse the anti-bacterial effects are and the broad range of diseases that are affected. Also listed in the table are some of the diseases these microorganisms can cause.[327] [328] [329]

---

[324] Haristoy X, Fahey J W, Scholtus I, Lozniewski A. Evaluation of antimicrobial effect of several isothiocyanates on *Helicobacter pylori*. *Planta Medica*. 2005;71: 326-330.
[325] Fahey J W, Haristoy X, Dolan P M, Kensler T W, Scholtus I, Stephenson K K, Talalay P, Lozniewski A. (2002) Sulforaphane inhibits extracellular, intracellular, and antibiotic-resistant strains of *Helicobacter pylori* and prevents benzo[*a*]pyrene-induced stomach tumors. *Proceedings of the National Academy of Sciences USA* 2002;99:p.7610-7615.
[326] http://www.emedicinehealth.com/helicobacter_pylori_h_pylori/articleem.htm#Overview
[327] Viera GH F, Mourão J A, Ângelo Â C, Costa R A, Viera R H. Antibacterial effect (in vitro) of Moringa oleifera and Annona muricata against Gram positive and Gram negative bacteria. *Rev Inst Med trop S Paulo*. 2010;May/June:
[328] Eilert U, Wolters B, Nahrstedt A. The antibiotic principle of seeds of *Moringa oleifera* and *Moringa stenopetala*. *Planta Medica* 1981;42: p.55-61.
[329] Jahn S A, Musnad H A, Burgstaller H., Tree that purifies water: Cultivating multipurpose Moringaceae in the Sudan. *Unasylva* 1986;38(152):p.23-28.

As a consequence of living on a polluted planet, we are being bombarded with environmental toxins and exposed to pathogenic bacteria.[330] We are at risk! When our physiological defense mechanisms cannot protect us, the immune, neurological and endocrine systems are jeopardized. A compromised immune system, demonstrated by decreased natural killer cell activity, is

TABLE III
Pathogenic Growth Inhibited or halted by
Moringa Oleifera

Pathogen	Diseases Caused by Pathogen	Researcher
Staphylococcus aureus	Pneumonia Eye infections Skin Infections Toxic shock syndrome Meningitis Food poisoning Osteomyelitis	Viera et al (2010)
Vibrio cholerae	Cholera	Viera et al (2010)
Escherichia coli	Food poisoning Urinary tract infection Diarrhoea Respiratory infections Wound infections	Viera et al (2010)
Salmonella Enteritidis	Food poisoning Diarrhoea	Viera et al (2010)
Mycobacterium phlei	Cardiac pacemaker	Eilert et al (1981)

---

[330]Crinnion W J. Environmental Medicine, Part 1: The Human Burden of Environmental Toxins and Their Common Health Effects. *Altern Med Rev*. 2000; 5(1):p52-63.

	infection	
Bacillus subtillis	Hypersensitivity pneumonitis Diarrhoea	Eilert et al (1981)
Serratia marcescens	Nosocomial infections Bacteremia Urinary tract infections	Jahn et al (1986)
Pseudomonas aeruginosa	Lung infection Pneumonia Skin infection Kidney infection Gastrointestinal infections Nosocomial infections	Jahn et al (1986)
Shigella	Dysentery	Jahn et al (1986)
Helicobacter pylori	Ulcers Chronic gastritis	Fahey et al (2002)

associated with a number of diseases such as cancer, autoimmune diseases and severe viral infections.[331] [332] [333] Compromised immune systems have a diminished immune cascade, (the immune response to an attack), and although there are many corollary pathways, none are as efficient as the cytokine pathways. When these pathways fail, a person suffers from chronic disease and this is the likely explanation. The body will be unable to accurately assess the scope, location and intensity of the threat and subsequently will not be capable of responding appropriately. Intervening in these areas of immune

---

[331] Whiteside T, Herberman R. The role of natural killer cells in human disease. Clin Immunology Immunopathology. 1989; 53: p1-23
[332] Spector GD et al. Immunodeficiency diseases and malignancy. Garden City Park, New York. The immunopathology of lymphoreticular neoplasms. Plenum Publishing. 1978; p203.
[333] Haschek W M, Rousseaux C G. Handbook of Toxicologic Pathology. San Diego. Academic Press. 1991.

deficits created by the aforementioned toxic threats will definitely reduce the risk of illness and disease. The immune system is generally the first to suffer.

ENHANCING THE IMMUNE SYSTEM

The self versus non-self protocol of the immune system is only as effective as the reliability of the various components of the immune system. Much research has been carried out investigating the level of natural killer (NK) cells and their role in predicting disease.[334] NK cells are the enforcers of the immune system, indiscriminately killing viruses, pathogenic intruders and cancer cells on sight.[335] Increased cytotoxic activity of lymphocytes enables the immune system to provide a more favorable response against any non-self intrusion including chronic diseases and cancer.[336] NK cells function even if the immune system cascade is compromised.

In a paper published by the University of Pittsburgh Cancer Institute titled, *Human NK Cells in Health and Disease*, the authors' findings were that increased NK cell activity amplified the body's resistance to cancer and viral infection and increased the body's ability to adapt to stress. Furthermore they found that increased NK cells activity optimized body function and increased the communication between the immune system, endocrine system and nervous system.[337] This will benefit those individuals with a

---

[334] Whiteside T, Herberman R. The role of natural killer cells in human disease. *Clin Immunology Immunopathology*. 1989;53:p.1-23.
[335] Simone C. Cancer & Nutrition. Garden City Park, New York. Avery Publishing Group. 1992; p45.
[336] Imai Kazue, Matsuyama Satoru et al. Natural cytotoxic activity of peripheral-blood lymphocytes and cancer incidence: an 11 year follow up study of a general population. Lancet. Vol 356 Issue 9244. November 2000; p1795-99.
[337] Whiteside T, Herberman R. Human natural killer cells in health and disease. Clin Immunotherapeutics. 1994; (1)1: p56-66.

suppressed immune response and also beneficially affect those with autoimmune disorders.

The unfortunate problem is that our current environment not only affects the ability of the immune system to function, but also the natural killer cell activity levels. Dr. Jesse Stoff, an immunologist from Arizona, found that the majority of the American population (98%) is functioning with only sixteen percent (16%) of the requisite number of natural killer cells considered to make up a strong immune system.[338] Several researchers have found a direct relationship between the number of these circulating lymphocytes and the risk of disease.[339] [340]

There are various nutrients that can have a beneficial effect on enhancing immune system function and *Moringa oleifera* certainly qualifies as one of these nutrients due to several phytonutrients.[341] [342] [343] Decreased dietary vitamin A levels have been shown to reduce the number of circulating natural killer cells and their function,

---

[338] Stoff J. An Examination of Immune Response Modulation in Humans by Antigen Infused Dialyzable Bovine Colostrum/Whey Extract Using A Double Blind Study. Tucson. Immune Consultants. 2001.
[339] Imai K, Matsuyama S, Miyake S, Suga K, et al. Natural cytotoxic activity of peripheral-blood lymphocytes and cancer incidence: an 11 year follow-up study of a general population. *Lancet*. 2000; 9244:p1795-1799.
[340] Whiteside T, Herberman R. The role of natural killer cells in human disease. *Clin Immunology Immunopathology*. 1989; 53:p1-23.
[341] Jayavardhanan K K, K Suresh K, Panikkar K R, Vasudevan D M. Modulatory potency of drumstick lectin on the host defense system. *Journal of Experimental Clinical Cancer Research* 1994;13(3):p.205-209
[342] Quisimbing *Medicinal Plants of the Philippines*. Katha Publishing Co Inc. Quezon City. 1978;p.346-349.
[343] Ramachandran C, Peter K V, Gopalakrishnan P K. 1980, Drumstick (Moringa oleifera): A multipurpose Indian Vegetable. *Economic Botany*, 34 (3) p.276-283.

predisposing the subjects to increased infection.[344] [345] Long-term beta-carotene supplementation enhances natural killer cell activity in elderly men, [346] decreasing the risk of infection and cancer. Several researchers have shown the effects of Moringa as a significant vitamin A and beta-carotene source.[347] [348] [349] [350] [351]

Researchers have determined that certain proteins, and polysaccharides found in various aspects of the Moringa tree act as immunomodulators and improve the function or enhance the immune system.[352] Mondal et al (2004) found that the bioactive glycosides called niaziridin and niazirin are derived from the leaves, pods, and bark of *Moringa oleifera.* [353] An immunoenhancing polysaccharide

[344] Dawson H D, Li N Q, Decicco K L, Nibert J A, Ross A C. Chronic marginal vitamin A status reduces natural killer cell number and function in aging Lewis rats. *J Nutr.* 1999; 129:p1510-1517.
[345] Bowman T A, Goonewardene M, Pasatiempo A M G, Ross A C, Taylor C E. Vitamin A deficiency decreases natural killer cell activity and interferon production in rats. *J. Nutr.* 1990; 120:p1264-1273.
[346] Santos M S, Meydani S N, Leka L, Wu D, Fotouli M et al. Natural killer cell activity in elderly men is enhanced by beta-carotene supplementation. *Am J Clin Nutr.* 1996; 64:p772-777.
[347] Geervani P, Devi A. Influence of protein and fat on the utilisation of carotene from drumstick (*Moringa oleifera*) leaves. *Indian J Med Res.* 1981;74:p.548-553.
[348] Delisle H, Bakari S, et al. Provitamin A content of traditional green leaves from Niger. *Cahiers Agricultures* 1997;6(6):p,553-560.
[349] Babu S C. Rural nutrition interventions with indigenous plant foods: a case study of vitamin deficiency in Malawi. International Food Policy Research Institute, Washington, DC. *Biotechnology, Agronomy Soc. Environ.* 2000 ;4(3):p.169-179.
[350] Nambiar V S, Seshadri S. Bioavailability trials of beta-carotene from fresh and dehydrated leaves of *Moringa oleifera* in a rat model. *Plant Foods for Human Nutrition.* 2001;56(1): 83-95.
[351] Fuglie L J. *The Miracle Tree: Moringa oleifera: Natural Nutrition for the Tropics*. Church World Service, Dakar. 1999;68pp.
[352] Randhawa G K, Kullar J S, Rajkumar. Bioenhancers from mother nature and their applicability in modern medicine. *Int J App Basic Med Res.* 2011;1:p.5-10.
[353] Mondal S, Chakraborty I, Pramanik M, Rout D, Islamm SS. Structural studies of an immunoenhancing polysaccharide isolated from

and niaziminin, which has the ability to inhibit tumor promoter-induced Epstein-Barr virus activation have been reported from the leaves of Moringa. [354] [355] [356] Any substance that can affect the part of the immune system known as the cytokine system is known as an immunomodulator. "Compounds that are capable of interacting with the immune system to upregulate or downregulate specific aspects of the host response can be classified as immunomodulators or biologic response modifiers."[357]

Immune modulation is repairing the damaged cytokine communication pathways while enhancing other aspects of the immune system. These repairs may include increasing production and activity levels of T cells, macrophages, natural killer cells leading to the subsequent production of interferon, interleukins and tumour necrotic factor. [358] These parameters are measurable indicators and the corresponding results will reveal the integrity of the cytokine pathway and consequently our immune system and our health. This ability to restore these proper levels holds a great deal of promise in allowing the body to deal

---

mature pods (fruits) of *Moringa oleifera* (Sajina). Med Chem Res 2004;13:p.390-□400.
[354] van der Hem L G, van der Vliet J A, Bocken C F, et al. Ling Zhi-8; studies of qa new immunomodulatring agent. *Transplantation*. 1995; 60(5): p438-443.
[355] Ooi V E, Liu F. Immunomodulation and anti-cancer activity of polysaccharide-protein complexes. *Curr Med Chem*. 2000; Jul: 7(7): p.715-729.
[356] Murakami A, Kitazono Y, Jiwajinda S, Koshimizu K, Ohigashi H. Niaziminin, a thiocarbamate from the leaves of *Moringa oleifera*, holds a strict structural requirement for inhibition of tumor-promoter-induced Epstein-Barr virus activation. *Planta Medica* 1998;64: p.319-323.
[357] Tzianabos A O. Polysaccharide Immunomodulators as Therapeutic Agents: Structural Aspects and Biologic Function. *Clinical Microbiology Reviews*. October 2000; 13;p523-533.
[358] Smith J E, Rowan N J, Sullivan R. Medicinal mushrooms: their therapeutic properties and current medical usage with special emphasis on cancer treatments. University of Strathclyde. 2002.

more favourably with allergic hypersensitivity and autoimmune disorders. Moringa contains the necessary nutrients to aid in the restoration of the immune system.[359]

Now what would happen if we could introduce a Moringa dietary regimen that affected a great many of these parameters and boosted immune system function?

---

[359] Jayavardhanan K K, K Suresh K, Panikkar K R, Vasudevan D M. Modulatory potency of drumstick lectin on the host defense system. *Journal of Experimental Clinical Cancer Research* 1994;13(3):p.205-209.

CHAPTER 5

MORINGA PROTEIN: FAR MORE THAN THE ESSENTIALS

"Corn is an efficient way to get energy calories off the land and soybeans are an efficient way of getting protein off the land, so we've designed a food system that produces a lot of cheap corn and soybeans resulting in a lot of cheap fast food."

Michael Pollan, Food Author

Humans have been described as nothing more than expressions of their protein. This of course refers to DNA and messenger RNA which determine exactly what the body builds. Think of your body as a nutritional bank. By making sufficient deposits, many transactions may be carried out each day. The importance of dietary protein has been somewhat underestimated by the general population and protein deficiency disorders such as kwashiorkor are a plague in countries where protein sources are diminished. Most people understand that muscle and tissue are made up of structural proteins and that DNA is a specific ordering of amino acids. How many people realize that protein: makes up our antibodies, controls the distribution of water between intracellular and extracellular compartments, transports hormones, provides nutrients and oxygen for tissues, buffers the plasma, and makes up blood clotting factors, enzymes, neurotransmitters and hormones? Individuals with protein deficiencies have weakened immune systems and may be predisposed to a number of diseases.[360] More importantly, the dietary deficiency of protein has a major impact on morbidity and mortality in children and infants suffering from inappropriate feeding habits.[361]

AMINO ACIDS

All proteins are made up of amino acids. Amino acids are composed of carbon, hydrogen, oxygen, nitrogen, and in some cases sulfur. Amino acids are one of the basic nitrogen-containing substances that go into the synthesis of all proteins in living matter. When dietary protein is digested, proteolytic enzymes separate the components (amino acids) which are then carried to the liver. There are twenty amino acids present in the human body and the liver manufactures about 80% of these. There are nine essential amino acids that must be received from dietary sources since the human body cannot synthesize them. The essential amino acids are: histidine, isoleucine, leucine, lysine, methionine, phenylalanine, threonine, tryptophan and valine. Histidine is essential for children and babies, not for adults. Very few foods, like *Moringa oleifera*, are known to contain all essential amino acids, hence, the importance of a complex, rich diet. As a matter of fact, Moringa is higher in amino acid content than legumes,[362] a source used by many vegetarians as their main protein source.

---

[360] Chandra R K. Nutrition, immunity and infection: present knowledge and future directions. Lancet. 1983; 1: p.688-691.
[361] WHO. Fifty-fifth World Health Assembly. Infant and Young Child Nutrition. Agenda Item 13.10. 18 May 2002.
[362] Abdulkarim S M, Long K, Lai O M, Muhammad S K S, Ghalazi H M. Some physic-chemical properties of Moringa oleifera seed oil extracted using solvent and aqueous enzymatic methods. *Food Chem.* 2005;93:p.253-263.

From personal experience I understand that it is important for vegetarians to ensure that their diet contains sufficient amounts of all the essential amino acids. Amino acids are subsequently sent to tissues where new cells are being created or sites where old damaged cells are being repaired. Amino acids are primarily absorbed in the small intestine, but small peptides, (groups of amino acids), are absorbed directly through the cell membranes and recombined into specially manufactured proteins.

In order for your body to function properly it needs to create over 40,000 specific proteins, (*Protein comes from the Greek word "first things."*), from singular amino acids, daily. Your body manufactures a diverse number of proteins that are responsible for a broad range of functions, (from bone growth to maintaining healthy biological terrain pH). Hemoglobin, is one of these complex proteins, which is responsible for carrying oxygen to all cells. Enzymes are also complex proteins and are necessary for all aspects of metabolism. Amino acids directly govern how the body works and functions.

The nutritional value of protein is determined by its amino acid content. This is why amino acids are called the building blocks of protein. Ingested proteins are hydrolyzed by the digestive system and then combined into the specific proteins needed for growth and to maintain good health. By supplying a more effective, bioavailable, nutritional amino acid source, we should be able to reverse or minimize the most of the life threatening effects of inadequate protein intake or absorption.

Protein deficiencies can lead to immune impairment, and increase susceptibility to infectious diseases. These, in turn, can cause or aggravate malnutrition as a result of many metabolic alterations. Immunoglobulins, antibodies, the complement system (after an invading organism is identified by antibodies the complement system breaks up the invading organism), and protease inhibitors are all proteins and may be effected to varying degrees. One of the problems with children suffering from protein-calorie malnutrition is that often there is not even a slight immune response to infection in these cases.[363]

Anemia can be caused by a deficiency of iron, protein, vitamin B12, folic acid, vitamin C, or copper. Anemia is common among children and the elderly. Low protein leads to decreased hemoglobin. It is estimated that more than 35% of the children and the elderly population experiences anemia. Among the most common symptoms of anemia are pallor, shortness of breath and fatigue.

Decreased lean body mass is a serious problem since protein is the fundamental building block that comprises muscles, organs, skeleton, antibodies, and enzymes. When lean body mass decreases, multiple functions including body movements, and breathing, can be seriously limited.

TABLE IV
AMINO ACIDS IN THE HUMAN BODY

Essential	Non-Essential
Isoleucine	Alanine
Leucine	**Asparagine**
Lysine	Aspartic acid
Methionine	Arginine
Phenylalanine	Cysteine
Threonine	Glutamine
Trytophan	Histidine
Valine	**Proline**
	Serine
	Tyrosine

[363] Smythe P M, Campbell J A H. The significance of bacteraemia of kwashiorkor. S Afr Med J. 1959; 33: p.777.

Increased body mass, such as obesity, is the most common form of malnutrition in North America (63% of the American population has been diagnosed as obese or overweight).[364] This form of malnutrition can cause or aggravate health disorders such as cardiovascular diseases, hypertension, shortness of breath, fatigue, or musculo-skeletal and neurological complications.

AMINO ACIDS IN *MORINGA OLEIFERA*

Isoleucine, an essential amino acid, builds proteins and enzymes, stimulates the brain, promotes muscle recovery after physical exercise, regulates blood sugar levels and is used to make the vital iron carrying hemoglobin.

Leucine is an essential amino acid used in the liver, but primarily in the muscle and fat. It is used in the bio-synthesis of sterols in the body and has the ability to stimulate muscle growth and inhibit muscular degradation.

Lysine, an essential amino acid, is important for proper growth, and it plays an essential role in the production of carnitine, a nutrient responsible for converting fatty acids into energy and helping to lower cholesterol. Lysine aids in the absorption of calcium, plays an important role in the formation of collagen, (benefits bones, connective tissues including skin, tendon, and cartilage) and the formation of antibodies, hormones and connective tissues.[365]

Methionine, one of the eight essential amino acids, is best known for its ability to supply sulfur and other compounds required for metabolism and growth. Sulfur is a key element and vital to the utilization of a number of

---

[364] http://www.cdc.gov/obesity/data/trends.html
[365] *Dietary Guidelines for Americans 2005*. Rockville, MD: US Dept of Health and Human Services and US Dept of Agriculture; 2005.

antioxidant nutrients. It lowers cholesterol and reduces fat in the liver while increasing lecithin production.

Phenylalanine is an essential amino acid that the body changes into tyrosine, another amino acid that is needed to make proteins, and neurotransmitters, including L-dopa, epinephrine, and norepinephrine, and thyroid hormones. Norepinephrine can affect mood, and different forms of phenylalanine have been proposed to treat depression.[366]

Threonine is an essential amino acid that helps the liver reduce fat, maintains protein balance and supports cardiovascular, liver, central nervous system, and immune system function by being involved in the production of antibodies. It is involved in the production of collagen, elastin, connective and muscle tissue, especially the heart, where it is found in a higher concentration and may decrease wound healing or recovery from injury. Links indicate that threonine may be beneficial in the treatment of Amyotrophic Lateral Sclerosis and Multiple Sclerosis.[367] [368]

Tryptophan is another of the essential amino acids for normal growth in infants and for nitrogen balance in adults.The body uses tryptophan to help make the B vitamin, niacin, and the neurotransmitter, serotonin. Serotonin regulates mood, appetite and sleep and decreased levels of this neurotransmitter is linked to depression. Trytophan supports your immune system, alleviates

---

[366] Birkmayer W, Riederer P, Linauer W, Knoll J. L-deprenyl plus l-phenylalanine in the treatment of depression. J Neural Trans. 1984;59(1):p.81-87.
[367] Roufs J B. L-threonine as a symptomatic treatment for amyotrophic lateral sclerosis (ALS). *Med Hypotheses*. 1991;34(1):p.20-23.
[368] Hauser S L, Doolittle T H, Lopez-Bresnahan M, Shahani B, Schoenfeld D, Shih V E, Grodon J, Lehrich J R. An antispatisticity effect of threonine in multiple sclerosis. *Arch Neurol*. 1992;49(9):p.923-926.

insomnia, reduces anxiety, depression, and relieves
symptoms of migraine headaches.[369]

Valine is an essential branched-chain amino acid
found in high concentration in muscle tissue. Valine has
been helpful in treating addictions. A deficiency may affect
the myelin covering of nerves. Aside from being a
component of many proteins, very little is known about the
independent functions of valine.[370]

Alanine is important when it comes to providing
energy for your muscle tissue, brain, and central nervous
system. This common amino acid is manufactured from
other metabolites in the liver and plays a key role in the
breakdown of glucose for energy and to stabilize serum
glucose levels during exercise. Alanine is used in the
production of neurotransmitters, antibodies and stimulates
lymphocyte production.[371]

Arginine plays an important role in cell division,
the healing of wounds, removing ammonia from the body,
immune function, and the release of hormones. It has been
shown in studies to cause the release of the growth
hormones considered necessary for muscle growth and
tissue repair, decreasing healing time.[372] Argenine is a
precursor for the production of nitric oxide and is related to
treating erectile dysfunction and providing cardiovascular

---

[369] Hartmann E. Effects of L-trytophan on sleepiness and on sleep. *J Psychiatric Res*. 1982-83;17(2):p.107-113.
[370] Haas, Elson M. *Staying Healthy With Nutrition: The Complete Guide to Diet and Nutritional Medicine*. Berkeley, California. Celestial Arts. 1992.
[371] Nelson D L, Cox M M. Principles of Biochemistry (4 ed.), New York. W H Freeman. 2005;p684-685.
[372] Stechmiller J K et al. Argenine supplementation and wound healing. *Nutrition in Clinical Practice*.2005;20(13):p.52-61.

benefits (lowering blood pressure)[373] as it relaxes smooth muscle, acts as a vasodilator and increases blood flow.[374]

Aspartic acid acts as a neurotransmitter and is involved in hormone production and release and nervous system function.[375]

Although *cysteine* is a non-essential amino acid, in certain cases such as premature infants, the elderly, or those with metabolic disease or a malabsorption syndrome it may be considered to be essential and must be supplied from dietary sources. Cysteine acts as an antioxidant and protects against radiation and pollution. Like all antioxidants, it will slow the aging process, deactivate free radicals, and neutralize toxins. Cysteine is involved in the formation of one the most potent detoxifiers in the body, glutathione in the lungs, liver, kidneys and bone marrow.

Glutamic acid is an amino acid that helps to prevent ammonia intoxication, and is an active neurotransmitter substance and is important for memory and learning.[376] By being converted into the anti-neurotransmitter GABA, glutamic acid may help to prevent seizures.[377]

Glycine is used for muscular tissue, DNA and RNA creation and converting glucose into energy. It prevents muscular degeneration by increasing levels of creatine. It is

---

[373] Gokce N. L-Argenine and hypertension. *J Nutrition*. 2004;134(10 Suppl):p.2807S-2811S.
[374] Andrew P J, Myer B. Enzymatic function of nitric oxide synthases. *Cardiovascular Research*. 1999;43(3):p.521-531.
[375] Lehninger A L, Nelson D L, Cox M M. *Principles of Biochemistry*. (3rd ed.) New York. W H Freeman. 2000.
[376] McEntee W, Crook T. Glutamate: Its role in learning, memory and the aging brain. *Psychopharmacology*. 1993;111(4):p.391-401.
[377] Sapolsky R. *Biology and Human Behavior: The Neurological Origins of Individuality*. (2nd ed.). The Teaching Company. 2005.

also important for the digestive system and nervous system function acting as an inhibitory neurotransmitter.[378]

Histidine is an amino acid that is essential in infants and may be essential for some adults.[379] Histidine is used to form histamine a neurological compound released during allergic responses. It is used for growth and for the repair of tissue, as well as the preservation of the myelin sheaths that protect nerve cells.[380] Histidine is required for the fabrication of both red and white blood cells, and helps to protect the body from damage caused by radiation and in heavy metals detoxification.

Serine plays a major role as a catalyst for many enzyme functions and synthesizes the fatty-acid based sheaths around nerve fibres. Serine is involved in the formation of immunoglobulins and antibodies strengthening the body's immune system. Plus, it synthesizes fatty acid sheaths around nerve fibers.

Proline, a non-essential amino acid, aids in the production of collagen and therefore affects joints, cartilage, tendons, the heart and skin.[381] It is a precursor to glutathione and very important for strengthening the heart.[382]

Tyrosine is a building block for several neurotransmitters, including epinephrine, norepinephrine,

---

[378] Nelson D L, Cox M M. *Principles of Biochemistry* (4th ed.). New York. W H Freeman. 2005;p 127,675-677,844,854.
[379] Kopple J D, Swendseid M E. Evidence that histidine is an essential amino acid in nbormal and chronically uremic man. *J Clin Invest.* 1975;55(5):p.881-891.
[380] Osiecki H, Meeke F, Smith J. *The Encyclopaedia of Clinical Nutrition- Volunme 1: The Nervous System.* BioConceps Publishing. Queensland. 2004.
[381] Balch P, Balch J. *Prescription for Nutrition* . Avery Books. New York.
[382] Null G. The complete encyclopedia of natural healing. Kebibgtim Publishing Corp. 1998.

and dopamine and supports the function of the thyroid, adrenal, and pituitary glands.[383] Tyrosine is a factor in regulating endocrine hormonal function and structurally is a component in most of the proteins in the body.

The virtually complete spectrum of amino acids in the 'drumstick tree'[384] indicates the potential capability to act as an ideal intervention regimen into any individual threatened by a protein deficiency. Children in third world countries on the brink of starvation suffer from kwashiorkor, a form of malnutrition that occurs when there is not enough protein in the diet, and Moringa has provided the solution to this for decades.[385] [386] [387] "Worldwide it is estimated that seven million people die each year from hunger-related causes, and the vast majority of these deaths are caused by chronic undernutrition." [388]

If *Moringa oleifera*, referred to as 'Nebeday" in Senegal is deemed to be the solution to a major malnutrition crisis in Africa, what benefits would be derived by a western population missing out on the majority of nutrients by eating a high-fructose based diet predisposing them to heart disease, cancer and diabetes?

---

[383] Meyers S. Use of neurotransmitter precursors for treatment of depression. *Altern Med Rev.* 2000;5(1):p.64-71.
[384] Paliwal R, Sharma V, Pracheta V. A review on Horse Radiah Tree (Moringa oleifera): A Multipurpose Tree with High Economic and Commercial Importance. *Asian Journal of Biotechnology.* 2011;3(4):p.317-328.
[385] Naidoo K K, Coopoosamy R M. Review on herbal remedies used by the 1860 South African Indian settlers. *African J Biotech.* 2011; 10 August:p. 8533-8538.
[386] Fahey J W. *Moringa oleifera*: a review of the medical evidence for its nutritional, therapeutic, and prophylactic properties. *Trees for Life Journal.* 2005;1(5) p. 1-13.
[387] Fuglie L J. Combating Malnutrition with Moringa. Development Potential for Moringa Products. *Church World Service.* Oct 29 to Nov 2, 2001.
[388] Church World Service, 1999. Facts have faces (brochure). New York.

CHAPTER 6

THE GOOD FATS ARE
NOT ONLY IN FISH

"If the doctors of today do not become the
nutritionists of tomorrow, then the nutritionists
of today will become the doctors of tomorrow."

Rockefeller Institute of Medicine research

There are four basic types of fat that the body takes
from food: cholesterol, saturated fat, mono-unsaturated fat
and polyunsaturated essential fatty acids. Nutritional
research has found that health is related to the type of fat
and not the amount of fat we consume. The polyunsaturated
essential fatty acids (PUFAs - Omega 3 [alpha-linolenic
acid] and Omega 6, [linoleic acid]) are the building blocks,
providing energy and being part of the structure of every
cell in our body. There is another type of fat that does not
originate in nature and that is the man-made hydrogenated
trans-fats that are found in just about all processed foods
containing shortening or oil. Saturated fats have been
linked to chronic diseases, inflammation, heart problems
and strokes.[389] Unsaturated fats nourish the body, and
confer protection against many diseases and fight
inflammation and infections.[390] Since the basis of this book
is to promote health, the focus will be on the good ones.

---

[389] Mayo Clinic. Dietary Fats: Know which ones to choose. 2011-02-
15. http://www.mayoclinic.com/health/fat/NU00262
[390] Yashodhara B M, Umakanth S, Pappachan J M, Bhat S K, Kamath
R, Choo B H. Omega-3 fatty acids: a comprehensive review of their
role in health and disease. *Postgrad Med J*. 2009;86(1000):p.84-90.

Omega-3 fatty acids are considered essential fatty acids because, like the amino acids that were discussed in the previous chapter, they are indispensable for human health. The body cannot make them and therefore we must ingest them from our diet. The fatty acids play a major role in the development of the brain and nervous system, maintaining cellular membrane integrity, and regulating blood pressure and clotting, just to name a few. Omega-3 fatty acids can be found in fish, such as salmon, tuna, and halibut, along with other seafood including algae and krill, some plants, nut oils and of course, *Moringa oleifera*.[391] [392] The omega fatty acids, sometimes referred to as polyunsaturated fatty acids (PUFAs), are involved in growth and brain function but they have become well known for reducing the risk of heart disease.[393] [394] The American Heart Association recommends eating fish twice a week, but they really are not aware of the complete nutritional package found in the 'drumstick tree.'[395]

Researchers have found that omega-3 fatty acids reduce inflammation and may help lower risk of the top life threatening chronic diseases: heart disease and cancer.[396] [397]

---

[391] Sena L P, Vanderjagt D J, Rivera C, Tsin A T C, Muhamadu I, Mahamadou O, Millson M, Pastuszyn A Glew R H. Analysis of nutritional components of the Republic of Niger. *Plant Foods for Human Nutrition*. 1998;52(1):p.17-30.

[392] Sánchez-Machado D I, Núñez-Gastélum J A, C, Reyes-Moreno C, Ramiréz-Wong B, López-Cervantes J. Nutritional quality of edible parts of Moringa oleifera. *Food Analytic Methods*. 2010;3(3)p.175-180.

[393] Angerer P, von Schacky C. n-3 polyunsaturated fatty acids and the cardiovascular system. *Curr Opin Lipidol*. 2000;11(1):p.57-63.

[394] Holman R T. The slow discovery of the importance of omega 3 essential fatty acids in human health. *J Nutr* 1998;128 (2 Suppl):p.427S–433S.

[395] Fahey J W. *Moringa oleifera*: a review of the medical evidence for its nutritional, therapeutic, and prophylactic properties. *Trees for Life Journal*. 2005;1(5) p. 1-13.

[396] Balk E M, Lichtenstein A H, Chung M et al. Effects of omega-3 fatty acids on serum markers of cardiovascular disease risk: A systematic review. *Atherosclerosis*. 2006;189(1):p.19-30.

[398] Omega-3 fatty acids are highly concentrated in neurological tissue, (especially the brain) and are significant for cognitive function and memory behavioral function.[399] Neonates, who do not get enough omega-3 fatty acids from their mothers during pregnancy, have an increased risk for vision and nerve problems. Symptoms of omega-3 fatty acid deficiency include fatigue, immune system weakness, poor memory, dry skin, hair loss, heart problems, eczema, memory loss, mood swings or depression, reproductive problems and poor circulation.

The dietary ratio of omega-3 and omega-6 is critical to optimal function.[400] Omega-3 fatty acids facilitate reduced inflammation, and conversely most omega-6 fatty acids tend to promote inflammation. The average American diet contains a disproportionate excess of omega-6 fatty acids (15:1) and may lead to inflammatory and cardiovascular disorders. The Mediterranean diet has a better ratio between the omega-3 and omega-6 fatty acids and consequently a far lower incidence of heart disease.[401] The Mediterranean diet includes foods rich in omega-3 fatty acids, including whole grains, fresh fruits, vegetables,

---

[397] Daniel C R, McCullough M L, Patel R C, Jacobs E J, Flanders W D, Thun M J, Calle E E. Dietary intake of omega-6 and omega-3 fatty acids and risk of colorectal cancer in a prospective cohort of U.S. men and women. *Cancer Epidemiol Biomarkers Prev.* 2009;18(2):p.516-525.
[398] Newcomer L M, King I B, Wicklund K G, Stanford J L. The association of fatty acids with prostate cancer risk. *Prostate.* 2001;47(4):p.262-268.
[399] Fotuhi M, Mohassel P, Yaffe K. Fish consumption, long-chain omega-3 fatty acids and risk of cognitive decline or Alzheimer disease: a complex association. *Nat Clin Pract Neurol.* 2009;5(3):p.140-152.
[400] Simopoulis A P. The importance of the ratio of omega-6/omega-3 essential fatty acids. *Biomedicine and Pharmacotherapy.* 2002;56:p.365-379.
[401] Kris-Etherton P, Eckel R H, Howard B V, St. Jeor S, Bazzare T L. AHA Science Advisory: Lyon Diet Heart Study. Benefits of a Mediterranean-style, National Cholesterol Education Program/American Heart Association Step I Dietary Pattern on Cardiovascular Disease. *Circulation.* 2001;103:p.1823.

fish, olive oil, garlic, as well as moderate wine consumption.

Moringa oleifera has an excellent source of omega-3 fatty acids and will counteract the usual disproportionate omega-3 to omega-6 ratio found in the average western diet.[402] [403] The proper ratio of Omega-6 to Omega-3 fatty acids is a key factor in preventing many of the modern chronic diseases including coronary heart disease, cardiac arrhythmias, high blood pressure, some types of cancer, and inflammatory and auto-immune disorders. There is a tremendous correlation between the health benefits attributed to the clinical research findings for the use of omega-3 fatty acid supplementation and Moringa.[404] [405] [406]

HYPERCHOLESTEROLEMIA

The presence of elevated levels of cholesterol in the blood has a direct relationship to cardiovascular disease, which is a major health risk in western diets.[407] Individuals

[402] Sena L P, Vanderjagt D J, Rivera C, Tsin A T C, Muhamadu I, Mahamadou O, Millson M, Pastuszyn A Glew R H. Analysis of nutritional components of the Republic of Niger. *Plant Foods for Human Nutrition*. 1998;52(1):p.17-30.

[403] Sánchez-Machado D I, Núñez-Gastélum J A, C, Reyes-Moreno C, Ramiréz-Wong B, López-Cervantes J. Nutritional quality of edible parts of Moringa oleifera. *Food Analytic Methods*. 2010;3(3)p.175-180.

[404] Fuglie L J. *The Miracle Tree: Moringa oleifera: Natural Nutrition for the Tropics*. Church World Service, Dakar. 1999;68pp.

[405] Fahey J W. *Moringa oleifera*: a review of the medical evidence for its nutritional, therapeutic, and prophylactic properties. *Trees for Life Journal*. 2005;1(5) p. 1-13.

[406] Fuglie L J. New uses of Moringa studied in Nicaragua. ECHO Development Notes #68, June, 2000.

[407] National Cholesterol Education Program (NCEP) Expert Panel on Detection, Evaluation, and Treatment of High Blood Cholesterol in Adults (Adult Treatment Panel, III) (2002-12-17). "Third Report of the National Cholesterol Education Program (NCEP) Expert Panel on Detection, Evaluation, and Treatment of High Blood Cholesterol in

following a Mediterranean diet have a propensity to have higher HDL (high density lipoprotein) or "good" cholesterol levels, which help promote heart health. HDL is able to strip away off arterial walls. Inuit Eskimos, whose diets are high in omega-3 fatty acids from their fatty 'cold water' fish diets, also tend to have increased HDL and decreased triglycerides (fats in the blood).[408] Fish oil and walnuts, (high in alpha linolenic acid or ANA, precursor to omega-3s), which reduce triglyceride levels have been reported to lower total cholesterol in people with elevated cholesterol levels.[409][410] *Moringa oleifera* has been shown to be a good source of omega-3 fatty acids and, although the mechanisms whereby the drumstick tree functions to decrease hypercholesterolemia are unknown, *Moringa oleifera* has been shown by several researchers to reduce serum cholesterol. [411][412][413][414][415]

Adults (Adult Treatment Panel III) final report." *Circulation*. 2002;106(25):p.3143-421.

[408]Dewailly E, Blanchet C, Lemieux S, et al. n-3 fatty acids and cardiovascular disease risk factors among the Inuit of Nunavik. *Am J Clin Nutr*. 2001;74(4):p.464-473.

[409] Mattar M, Obeid O. Fish oil and the management of hypertriglyceridemia. *Nutr Health*. 2009;20(1):p.41-9.

[410] Kris-Etherton P, Eckel RH, Howard BV, St. Jeor S, Bazzare TL. AHA Science Advisory: Lyon Diet Heart Study. Benefits of a Mediterranean-style, National Cholesterol Education Program/American Heart Association Step I Dietary Pattern on Cardiovascular Disease. *Circulation*. 2001;103:p.1823.

[411] Ghasi S, Nwobodo E, Ofili J O. Hypocholesterolemic effects of crude extract of leaf of *Moringa oleifera* Lam in high-fat diet fed Wistar rats. *J Ethnopharmacology* 2000 ;69(1):p.21-25.

[412] Gilani A H, Aftab K, Suria A, Siddiqui S, Saleem R, Siddiqui B S, Faizi S. Pharmacological studies on hypotensive and spasmolytic activities of pure compounds from *Moringa oleifera*. *Phytotherapy Research* 1994;8(2):p.87-91.

[413] Mehta L K, Balaraman R, Amin A H, Bafna P A , Gulati O D. (2003) Effect of fruits of *Moringa oleifera* on the lipid profile of normal and hypocholesterolaemic rabbits. *J Ethnopharmacology* 2003;86:p.191-195.

[414] Dahot M U, Memon A R. Properties of *Moringa oleifera* seed lipase. *Pakistan Journal of Scientific and Industrial Research* 1987;30(11):p.832-835.

HIGH BLOOD PRESSURE (Hypertension)

Several clinical studies suggest that diets rich in omega-3 fatty acids lower blood pressure in people with hypertension. A meta-analysis of seventeen clinical studies using fish oil supplements found that subjects ingesting between three and five and a half grams of fish oil daily were able to reduce blood pressure if they were not already on medication for hypertension.[416] [417] [418] [419] [420] It is quite important for all readers of this book to take into consideration that it was also noted in this analysis that dosages of fish oil of this magnitude should only be taken under the care of a qualified physician.

The leaves and the pods of the Moringa tree have been demonstrated to reduce blood pressure as well. [421] [422]

---

[415] Chumark P, Khunawat P, Sanvarinda Y, Phornchirasilp S, Morales N P, Phivthong-ngam L, Ratanachamnong P, Srisawat S, Pongrapeeporn K-S. The in vitro and ex vivo antioxidant properties, hypolipidaemic and antiatherosclerotic activities of water extract of Moringa oleifera Lam. leaves. J Ethnopharmacology. 2008; 116:p.439-446.

[416] Appel L J, Miller E R , Seidler A J, et al. Does supplementation of diet with 'fish oil' reduce blood pressure? A meta-analysis of controlled clinical trials. Arch Intern Med. 1993;153:p.1429–1438.

[417] Mori T A, Watts G F, Burke V, et al. Differential effects of eicosapentaenoic acid and docosahexaenoic acid on vascular reactivity of the forearm microcirculation In hyperlipidemic, overweight men. Circulation. 2000;102: p.1264–1269.

[418] Mori T A. Omega-3 fatty acids and blood pressure. Cell Mol Biol (Nosiy-le-grand). 2010;56(1):p.83-92.

[419] Morris M C, Sacks F, Rosner B. Does fish oil lower blood pressure? A meta-analysis of controlled trials. Circulation. 1993;88:p.523–533.

[420] Howe P R. Dietary fats and hypertension: focus on fish oil. Ann N Y Acad Sci. 1997;827:p.339–352.

[421] Faizi S, Siddiqui BS, Saleem R, Siddiqui S, Aftab K, Gilani AH. Fully acetylated carbamates and hypotensive thiocarbamate glycosides from Moringa oleifera. Phytochemistry 1995;38:957-63.

[422] Tabassum N, Ahmad F. Role of natural herbs in the treatment of hypertension. 2011;5:p.30-40.

[423] [424] [425] [426] [427] [428] [429] [430] Although, due to the lack of research into the mechanisms, the means of the blood pressure reduction is unknown. However the results are the same, decreased hypertension.

HEART DISEASE

The function of omega-3 fatty acids in cardiovascular disease has been well established.[431] One of the best ways to help prevent heart disease is to eat a diet low in saturated fat and to eat foods that contain good amounts of in monounsaturated and polyunsaturated fats

---

[423] Saleem R, Meinwald J. Synthesis of novel hypotensive aromatic thiocarbamate glycosides. *Journal of the Chemical Society Perkins Transactions*. 2000;1: 391-394.

[424] Fuglie L J. *The Miracle Tree: Moringa oleifera: Natural Nutrition for the Tropics*. Church World Service, Dakar. 1999;68pp.

[425] Faizi S, Siddiqui B S, Saleem R, Aftab K, Shaheen F, Gilani A H. Hypotensive constituents from the pods of *Moringa oleifera*. *Planta Medica* 1998;64:p.225-228.

[426] Faizi S, Siddiqui B S, Saleem R, Aftab K, Shaheen F, Gilani A H. Fully acetylated carbamate and hypotensive thiocarbamate glycosides from *Moringa oleifera*. *Phytochemistry* 1995;38:p.957-963.

[427] Faizi S, BS Siddiqui, et al. Isolation and structure elucidation of novel hypotensive agents, niazinin A, niazinin B, niazimicin and niaziminin A plus B from *Moringa oleifera*: The first naturally occurring thiocarbamates. *Journal of the Chemical Society Perkin Transactions*. 1992;I(23):p.3237-3241.

[428] Faizi S, et al. Novel hypotensive agents, niazimin A, niazimin B, niazicin A and niazicin B from *Moringa oleifera*: Isolation of first naturally occurring carbamates. *Journal of the Chemical Society Perkin Transactions I:* 1994;p.3035-3040.

[429] Faizi S, Siddiqui B S, Saleem R, Aftab K, Shaheen F, Gilani A H. Isolation and structure elucidation of new nitrile and mustard oil glycosides from *Moringa oleifera* and their effect on blood pressure. *Journal of Natural Products* 1994;57:p.1256-1261.

[430] Gilani A H, Aftab K, Suria A, Siddiqui S, Saleem R, Siddiqui B S, Faizi S. Pharmacological studies on hypotensive and spasmolytic activities of pure compounds from *Moringa oleifera*. *Phytotherapy Research* 1994;8(2):p.87-91.

[431] Balk E M, Lichtenstein A H, Chung M et al. Effects of omega-3 fatty acids on serum markers of cardiovascular disease risk: A systematic review. Atherosclerosis. 2006;189(1):p.19-30.

(including omega-3 fatty acids). Clinical evidence suggests that omega-3 fatty acids help reduce risk factors for heart disease, including high cholesterol and high blood pressure. [432] [433] As we have seen in the previous chapter and previous paragraphs, Moringa does this as well. Omega fatty acids have been shown to lower levels of triglycerides (fats in the blood), and to decrease the risk and incidence of death, heart attack,[434] stroke,[435] abnormal heart rhythms (in previous heart attack sufferers) and seems to prevent and treat atherosclerosis by inhibiting the development of plaque and blood clots.[436] [437] [438] Although there has not been a direct investigation into Moringa and cardiovascular disease, many of the vitamin and phytonutrient parameters associated with   beneficial effects for this condition (antioxidants, beta carotene, vitamin C, vitamin E, omega fatty acids) are supplied by this fast growing, hardy micronutrient storehouse.[439]

---

[432] Calo L, Bianconi L, Colivicchi F et al. N-3 Fatty acids for the prevention of atrial fibrillation after coronary artery bypass surgery: a randomized, controlled trial. *J Am Coll Cardiol*. 2005;45:p.1723-1728.
[433] Galli C, Risé P. Fish consumption, omega 3 fatty acids and cardiovascular disease. The science and the clinical trials. *Nutr Health*. 2009;20(1):11-20.
[434] de Lorgeril M, Salen P, Martin J L, et al. Mediterranean diet, traditional risk factors, and the rate of cardiovascular complications after myocardial infarction: final report of the Lyon Diet Heart Study. *Circulation*. 1999;99:p.779–785.
[435] Simon J A, Fong J, Bernert J T Jr, et al. Serum fatty acids and the risk of stroke. *Stroke*. 1995;26:p.778–782.
[436] Calo L, Bianconi L, Colivicchi F et al. N-3 Fatty acids for the prevention of atrial fibrillation after coronary artery bypass surgery: a randomized, controlled trial. *J Am Coll Cardiol*. 2005;45:p.1723-1728.
[437] Angerer P, von Schacky C. n-3 polyunsaturated fatty acids and the cardiovascular system. *Curr OpinLipidol*. 2000;11(1):p.57-63.
[438] Boelsma E, Hendriks HF. Roza L. Nutritional skin care: health effects of micronutrients and fatty acids. *Am J Clin Nutr*. 2001;73(5):p.853-864.
[439] Fahey J W. *Moringa oleifera*: a review of the medical evidence for its nutritional, therapeutic, and prophylactic properties. *Trees for Life Journal*. 2005;1(5) p. 1-13.

DIABETES

As a general rule, people suffering from diabetes often have high triglyceride and low HDL levels. Omega-3 fatty acids, in proper proportions, can help lower triglycerides and apoproteins (markers of diabetes), and raise HDL, so therefore a diet containing the proper ratio of essential fatty acids may help people with diabetes.[440] [441] Norris et al (2007) found that a dietary intake of omega-3 fatty acids is associated with reduced risk in children at increased genetic risk for type 1 diabetes.[442] Brostow et al (2011) found a similar decreased risk of type 2 diabetes with omega-3 fatty acids.[443] *Moringa oleifera* has been shown to demonstrate anti-diabetic and hypoglycemic (reducing serum glucose levels) combating the effects of diabetes. [444] [445] [446] [447] Perhaps the plentiful supply of

---

[440] Krishna Mohan I, Das UN. Prevention of chemically induced diabetes mellitus in experimental animals by polyunsaturated fatty acids. *Nutrition*. 2001; 17(2):126-151.

[441] Benhamou P Y, Mullen Y, Clare-Salzer M, et al. Essential fatty acid deficiency prevents autoimmune diabetes in non-obese diabetic mice through a positive impact on antigen-presenting cells and Th2 lymphocytes. *Pancreas*. 1995;11(1):p.26-37.

[442] Norris J, Yin X, Lamb M M, Barriga K, Seifert J, Hoffman M, Orton H D, Baron A E, Clare-Salzler M, Chase H P, Szabo N J, Erlich H, Eisenbarth G S, Rewers M. Omega-3 polyunsaturated fatty acid intake and island autoimmunity in children at increased risk for type I diabetes. *JAMA*. 2007;298(12):p.1420-1428.

[443] Brostow D P, Odegaard A O, Koh W P, Duval S, Gross M D, Yuan J M, Pereira M A. Omega-3 fatty acids and incident type 2 diabetes: the Singapore Chinese Health Study, 2011;94(2):p.520-526.

[444] Asres K. The major constituents of the acetone fraction of Ethiopian *Moringa stenopetala* leaves. *Mansoura Journal of Pharmacological Science*. 1995;11(1):p.55-64.

[445] Faizi S, Siddiqui B S, Saleem R, Aftab K, Shaheen F, Gilani A H. Bioactive Compounds from the leaves and pods of *Moringa oleifera*. *New Trends in Natural Products Chemistry* 1998;p.175-183.

[446] Kar A, Choundhary B, Bandyopadhyay N. Preliminary studies on the inorganic constituents of some indigenous hypoglycaemic herbs on oral glucose tolerance test, *J Ethnopharmacology*. 1999;64(2):p.179-184.

omega-3 fatty acids in Moringa[448] is responsible for these effects.[449] [450]

ARTHRITIS

Many of the clinical studies conducted examining the relationship between omega-3 fatty acids and arthritis have focused primarily on rheumatoid arthritis (RA).[451] [452] RA is a chronic, systemic inflammatory autoimmune disease that may affect many tissues and organs, but principally attacks synovial joints causing pain and swelling in the joints. A number of studies have found that omega-3 fatty acids help reduce symptoms of RA, including, inflammation, joint pain and morning stiffness.[453] [454] [455] Galarraga et al (2008) found that people with RA who take n-3 fatty acids were able to lower their dose of non-steroidal anti-inflammatory drugs (NSAIDs),

---

[447] Makonnen E, Hunde A, Damecha G. Hypoglycaemic effect of *Moringa stenopetala* aqueous extract in rabbits. *Phytotherapy Research* 1997;11:p.147-148
[448] Anhwange B A, Ajibola V O, Oniye S J. Chemical studies of the seeds of Moringa oleifera(Lam) and Detarium microcarpum (Guill and Sperr). *J Biological Sci*. 2004;4:p.711-715.
[449] Paliwal R, Sharma V, Pracheta V. A review on Horse Radiah Tree (Moringa oleifera): A Multipurpose Tree with High Economic and Commercial Importance. *Asian J Biotechnology*. 2011;3(4):p.317-328.
[450] Anwar F, Latif S, Ashraf M, Gilani A H. Moringa oleifera: A food plant with multiple medicinal uses. *Phytother Res*. 2007;21:p.17-25.
[451] Berbert A A, Kondo C R, Almendra C L et al. Supplementation of fish oil and olive oil in patients with rheumatoid arthritis. *Nutrition*. 2005;21:p.131-136.
[452] Hagen K B, Byfuglien MG, Falzon L, Olsen SU, Smedslund G. Dietary interventions for rheumatoid arthritis. *Cochrane Database Syst Rev*. 2009; Jan 21;(1):CD006400.
[453] Kremer J M. N-3 fatty acid supplements in rheumatoid arthritis. *Am J Clin Nutr*. 2000;(suppl 1)p.349S-351S.
[454] Ruggiero C, Lattanzio F, Lauretani F, et al. Omega-3 polyunsaturated fatty acids and immune-mediated dieases: inflammatory bowel disease and rheumatoid arthritis. *Curr Pharm Des*. 2009;15(36):p.4135-4138.
[455] Sales C, Oliviero F, Spinella P. The Mediterranean diet model in inflammatory rheumatic diseases. *Reumatismo*. 2009;61(1):p.10-14.

but it does not appear to slow progression of RA, only to treat the symptoms and damage to the synovial membranes of the joint continues.[456] Bahadori et al (2010) found that oral supplementation of omega-3 fatty acids lengthens the benefits of this therapeutic approach in the treatment of arthritis.[457] A study by Curtis (2002) indicated that diets rich in omega-3 fatty acids (and low in the inflammatory omega-6 fatty acids) was able to help rebuild cartilage and help people with osteoarthritis (degenerative arthritis). [458] A further study on osteoarthritis (Zainal 2009) found that there were benefits to be derived from increasing intake of omega-3 fatty acids. [459]

One of the most impressive studies that actually links Moringa to derived benefits was the meta-analysis conducted by Goldberg et al (2007). "The results suggest that omega-3 PUFAs are an attractive adjunctive treatment for joint pain associated with rheumatoid arthritis, inflammatory bowel disease, and dysmenorrhea."[460] Moringa is a rich dietary source of omega-3 PUFAs.[461] [462]

---

[456] Galarraga B, Ho M, Youssef H M, et al. Cod liver oil (n-3 fatty acids) as an non-steroidal anti-inflammatory drug sparing agent in rheumatoid arthritis. *Rheumatology* (Oxford) 2008;47(5):p.665-669.
[457] Bahadori B, Uitz E, Thonhofer R, et al. omega-3 fatty acids infusions as adjuvant therapy in rheumatoid arthritis. *JPEN J Parenter Enteral Nutr*. 2010;34(2):p.151-5.
[458] Curtis C L, Rees S G, Little C B, et al. Pathologic indicators of degradation and inflammation in human osteoarthritic cartilage are abrogated by exposure to n-3 fatty acids. *Arthritis Rheum*. 2002;46(6):p.1544-1553.
[459] Zainal Z, Longman AJ, Hurst S, et al. Relative efficacies of omega-3 polyunsaturated fatty acids in reducing expression of key proteins in a model system for studying osteoarthritis. *Osteoarthritis Cartilage*. 2009;17(7):p.896-905.
[460] Goldberg R J, Katz J. A meta-analysis of the analgesic effects of omega-3 polyunsaturated fatty acid supplementation for inflammatory joint pain. *Pain*. 2007; May 29L1-2):p.210-223.
[461] Anhwange B A, Ajibola V O, Oniye S J. Chemical studies of the seeds of Moringa oleifera(Lam) and Detarium microcarpum (Guill and Sperr). *J Biological Sci*. 2004;4:p.711-715.

When looking at arthritis from a diversity of perspectives, Moringa has been used to treat the pain and inflammatory conditions caused by arthritis, a disorder affecting nearly forty million Americans and other degenerative diseases. [463] [464] [465] [466] [467] [468] [469]

OSTEOPOROSIS

Every three seconds somewhere on earth, an osteoporotic induced fracture occurs.[470] More than two hundred million women around the world suffer from osteoporosis.[471] Some studies (Kruger et al 1997) suggest that omega-3 fatty acids may help increase levels of

---

[462] Paliwal R, Sharma V, Pracheta V. A review on Horse Radiah Tree (Moringa oleifera): A Multipurpose Tree with High Economic and Commercial Importance. *Asian Journal of Biotechnology*. 2011;3(4):p.317-328.

[463] Fuglie L J. *The Miracle Tree: Moringa oleifera: Natural Nutrition for the Tropics*. Church World Service, Dakar. 1999:68pp.

[464] Anwar F, Latif S, Ashraf M, Gilani A H. Moringa oleifera: A food plant with multiple medicinal uses. *Phytother Res*. 2007;21:p.17-25.

[465] Delaveau P, et al. Oils of Moringa oleifera and Moringa drouhardii. *Plantes Médicinales et Phytothérapie*. 1980;14(10):p.29-33.

[466] Caceres A, Saravia A, Rizzo S, Zabala L, Leon E D, Nave F. Pharmacological properties of Moringa oleifera. 2: Screening for antispasmodic, anti-inflammatory and diuretic activity. *J Ethnopharmacol*. 1992;36:p.233-237.

[467] Ezeamuzie I C, Ambakederemo A W, Shode F O, Ekwebelm S C. Antiinflammatory effects of *Moringa oleifera* root extract. *Int J Pharmacog*. 1996;34(3):p.207-212.

[468] Rao K N V, Gopalakrishnan V, Loganathan V, Shanmuganathan S. Antiinflammatory activity of Moringa oleifera Lam. *Ancient Science of Life*. 1999;18(3-4):p.195-198.

[469] Udapa S L, Udapa A L, et al. Studies on the anti-inflammatory and wound healing properties of Moringa oleifera and Aegle marmelos. *Fitoterapia*. 1994;65(2):p.119-123.

[470] Johnell O, Kanis J A. An estimate of the worldwide prevalence and disability associated with osteoporotic fractures. Osteoporos Int. 2006; 17:p.1726.

[471] Kanis J A. *WHO Technical Report*, University of Sheffield, UK. 2007:p.66

calcium in the body and improve bone strength.[472]   To reiterate what we stated in an earlier chapter, the hallmark of osteoporosis is characterized by low bone mass and micro-architectural   deterioration   of   bone   tissue.[473] Essential fatty acids do not have a predominant place in the literature regarding osteoporosis, but studies have shown the fatty acids to increase calcium absorption by augmenting the effects of vitamin D. This reduces the urinary excretion of calcium and increases the calcium that is deposited in the bone matrix, stimulating the creation of collagen.[474] The Kruger study also identifies that dietary deficiencies of essential fatty acids create greater risk for bone loss and calcification of other tissues and blood vessels than those with normal levels of these fatty acids.[475] In a study of women over 65 with osteoporosis, those who took EFA supplements had less bone loss over three years than those who took placebo. Many of these women also experienced an increase in bone density.[476] Maggio et al (2009) suggests that dietary fats (omega 3) have a positive effect on decreasing bone loss.[477]   It has already been established that *Moringa oleifera* provides much needed omega-3 fatty acids,[478] but it also provides more than ample quantities of calcium, magnesium, Vitamin D and

---

[472] Kruger M, Horrobin D. Calcium metabolism, osteoporosis and essential fatty acids: a review. *Prog Lipid Res*.1997;36(2-3):131-151.
[473] Brunader R, Shelton D K. Radiologic Bone Assessment in the Evaluation of Osteoporosis. *Am Fam Physician*. 2002; p1357-1364.
[474] Kruger M, Horrobin D. Calcium metabolism, osteoporosis and essential fatty acids: a review. *Prog Lipid Res*. 1997;36(2-3):p.131-151.
[475] Kruger M, Horrobin D. Calcium metabolism, osteoporosis and essential fatty acids: a review. *Prog Lipid Res*.1997;36(2-3):131-151.
[476] Agnusdei D, Crepaldi G, Isaia G, et al. A double blind, placebo-controlled trial of ipriflavone for prevention of postmenopausal spinal bone loss. *Calcif Tissue Int*. 1997;61:p.142-147.
[477] Maggio M, Artoni A, Lauretani F, Borghi L, Nouvenne A, Valenti G, Ceda G P. The impact of omega-3 fatty acids on osteoporosis. *Curr Pharm Des*. 2009;15(36):p.4157-4164.
[478]Paliwal R, Sharma V, Pracheta V. A review on Horse Radiah Tree (Moringa oleifera): A Multipurpose Tree with High Economic and Commercial Importance. *Asian Journal of Biotechnology*. 2011;3(4):p.317-328.

zinc; nutrients needed for calcium absorption and strengthening bone matrix.[479 480 481 482 483 484]

ADD & ADHD
(Attention Deficit/hyperactivity disorder)

Attention deficit disorder is characterized by symptoms displayed by subjects which include poor attention span, impulsivity, distractibility, increased motor activity, and poor social skills. These disorders are part of the autism spectrum. Toxins such as mercury, lead, pesticides, and in utero smoking exposure lead to higher of autism and/or ADHD.[485]

It is postulated that children with attention deficit/hyperactivity disorder (ADHD) may have decreased levels of certain essential fatty acids.[486] In a 2002

---

[479] Babu S C. Rural nutrition interventions with indigenous plant foods: a case study of vitamin deficiency in Malawi. International Food Policy Research Institute, Washington, DC. *Biotechnology, Agronomy Soc. Environ.* 2000;4(3) :p.169-179.

[480] Fuglie L J. *The Miracle Tree: Moringa oleifera: Natural Nutrition for the Tropics.* Church World Service, Dakar. 1999;68 pp.

[481] Fahey J W. *Moringa oleifera*: a review of the medical evidence for its nutritional, therapeutic, and prophylactic properties. *Trees for Life Journal.* 2005;1(5) p. 1-13.

[482] Pankaja N, Prakash J.(1994) Availability of calcium from kilkeerai (*Amaranthus tricolor*) and drumstick (*Moringa oleifera*) greens in weanling rats. *Nahrung* 1994;38:p.199-203.

[483] Barminas J T, Charles M, Emmanuel D. Mineral composition of non-conventional leafy vegetables. *Plant Foods for Human Nutrition* Dordrecht 1998;53(1):p.29-36.

[484] Price M L. *The Moringa Tree*. ECHO Technical Note. Educational Concerns for Hunger Organization. N. Ft. Meyers, FL. 1985.

[485] Curtis L T, Patel K. Nutritional and environmental approaches to preventing and treating autism and attention deficit hyperactivity disorder (ADHD): a review. *J Altern Complement Med.* 2008; 2008;14(1):p.79-85.

[486] Burgess J, Stevens L, Zhang W, Peck L. Long-chain polyunsaturated fatty acids in children with attention-deficit hyperactivity disorder. *Am J Clin Nutr.* 2000;71(suppl):p.327S-330S.

University of Maryland clinical study of nearly 100 boys, those with lower levels of omega-3 fatty acids had more learning and behavioral problems (such as temper tantrums and sleep disturbances) than boys with normal omega-3 fatty acid levels. More research is necessary, but including foods that are high in omega-3 fatty acids is a reasonable strategy for someone with ADHD.[487] *Moringa oleifera* is an excellent dietary source of omega 3 fatty acids and is a nutritional pharmacopeia. Current theories for a non-pharmaceutical regimen indicate nutritional support and detoxification of heavy metals and chemical toxins. ADD and ADHD are extremely complex conditions in which nutritional and environmental factors play major roles.[488] The nutritional impact of *Moringa oleifera* suggests that it should become part of the dietary regimen in those affected by any aspect of the autistic spectrum.[489 490 491 492]

COGNITIVE FUNCTION

Many studies show that reduced intake of omega-3 fatty acids is associated with an increased risk of age related decline in cognitive function including both dementia, and Alzheimer's disease. Scientists believe the

---

[487] Aben A, Danckaerts M. Omega-3 and omega-6 fatty acids in the treatment of children and adolescents with ADHD. *Tijdschr Psychiatr*.2010;52(2):p.89-97.

[488] Curtis L T, Patel K. Nutritional and environmental approaches to preventing and treating autism and attention deficit hyperactivity disorder (ADHD): a review. *J Altern Complement Med*. 2008; 2008;14(1):p.79-85.

[489] Dahot M U, Memon A R. Nutritive significance of oil extracted from *Moringa oleifera* seeds. *Journal of Pharmacy of the University of Karachi* 1985;3(2):p.75-80.

[490] Dhar B, Gupta O P. Nutritional value of Shigru (Moringa oleifera Lam). *B M E B R*. 1982;3(2-4):p.280-288.

[491] Freiberger C E, Vanderjagt D J, et al. Nutrient content of the edible leaves of seven wild plants from Niger. *Plant Foods for Human Nutrition* 1998;53(1): 57-69.

[492] Reddy N S, Bhatt G. Contents of minerals in green leafy vegetables cultivated in soil fortified with different chemical fertilizers. *Plant Foods for Human Nutrition*. 2001;56:p.1-6.

omega-3 fatty acid DHA is protective against Alzheimer's disease and dementia.[493] In individuals with Alzheimer's Disease, dementia, or cognitive impairment, low levels of n-3 fatty acids may be a risk factor for cognitive impairment and/or dementia.[494] Moringa has also been shown to benefit those with cognitive function deficits, dementia and Alzheimer's Disease.[495 496]

---

[493] Cole GM. Omega-3 fatty acids and dementia. *Prostaglandins Leukot Essent Fatty Acids.* 2009; 81(2-3):p.213-21.

[494] Conquer J A, Tierney M C, Zecevic J, Bettger W J, Fisher R H. Fatty acid analysis of blood plasma of patients with Alzheimer's disease other types of dementia and cognitive impairment. *Lipids.* (2000);35:1301-1312.

[495] Obulesu O, Rao D M. Effect of plant extracts on Alzheimer's disease: An insight into therapeutic avenues. *J Neurosciences in Rural Practice.* 2011;2(1):p.56-61.

[496] Ganguly R, Hazra R, Ray K, Guha D. Effect of Moringa oleifera in experimental model of Alzheimer's disease: Role of antioxidants. *Ann Neurosci.* 2005;12:p.36-9.

CHAPTER 7

LOOKING AT THE BIG PICTURE

"It is health that is the real wealth
and not pieces of gold and silver".

Mahatma Gandhi

By now we must realize that no matter which of the hundreds of names we use for Moringa, it is probably one of if not the most dynamic phytonutrient rich plant on this planet. If we look only at the folklore and the messages being handed down through the generations, this tree has amazing abilities to effect a broad spectrum of maladies. This fact should tell us that the vitamins, minerals and diverse phytonutrients are indeed quite bioavailable. Hippocrates issued the message more than two thousand years ago, "Let your food be your medicine and your medicine be your food" and this was millennia before he actually knew how many additives we were going to add and just how badly we were going to destroy the nutritional value of our food.

For those seeking health, we just have to examine some real facts to determine what credibility Moringa has. If we look at the raw food movement, we can see the shift away from adulterating the food we eat and a new folklore being created. Some of the diseases that plague mankind now are simply disappearing by diet alone.

Dr. Gabriel Cousens, a holistic medical doctor in practice for almost forty years, has found that switching to a raw food diet works to significantly reduce serum glucose levels and can effectively eliminate type II diabetes in about a month.[497] There are also dynamic effects on type I diabetes. As was stated earlier in this book, according to the 2011 National Diabetes Fact Sheet, 8.3% of the American public has diabetes and that does not take into effect the 79,000,000 people who are pre-diabetic.[498] Now let's shift the focus back to Moringa, a tree that has demonstrated the mechanisms that lead to the decrease of serum glucose.[499] [500] [501] [502] [503]

The Gerson diet, introduced by Dr. Max Gerson in 1945, is a non-specific dietary regimen that effectively treats many different conditions by healing the body as a whole, rather than selectively targeting a specific condition or symptom, and doing it by means of nutritional intervention. For more than the last half century, thousands of people who were suffering from assorted cancers, heart disease, diabetes, arthritis and autoimmune disorders have seen these symptoms vanish and either go into total remission or may be considered cured. The theory behind this therapy is to "support each important metabolic requirement by flooding the body with nutrients."[504]

---

[497] Cousens G. There Is a Cure for Diabetes: The Tree of Life 21-Day+ Program. North Atlantic Books, Berkeley, CA. 2008;446pp.

[498] http://www.diabetes.org/diabetes-basics/diabetes-statistics/

[499] Asres K. The major constituents of the acetone fraction of Ethiopian *Moringa stenopetala* leaves. *Mansoura Journal of Pharmacological Science*. 1995;11(1):p.55-64.

[500] Faizi S, Siddiqui B S, Saleem R, Aftab K, Shaheen F, Gilani A H. Bioactive Compounds from the leaves and pods of *Moringa oleifera*. *New Trends in Natural Products Chemistry* 1998;p.175-183.

[501] Kar A, Choundhary B, Bandyopadhyay N. Preliminary studies on the inorganic constituents of some indigenous hypoglycaemic herbs on oral glucose tolerance test. *J Ethnopharmacology*. 1999;64(2):p.179-184.

[502] Kar A, Choundhary B, Bandyopadhyay N. Comparative evaluation of hypoglycaemic activity of some Indian medicinal plants in alloxan diabetic rats. *J Ethnopharmacol*. 2003;Jan; 84 (1):p.105-108.

[503] Makonnen E, Hunde A, Damecha G. Hypoglycaemic effect of *Moringa stenopetala* aqueous extract in rabbits. *Phytotherapy Research* 1997;11:p.147-148

[504] http://gerson.org/GersonTherapy/gersontherapy.htm

When we examine the preceding examples, we should now pay more heed to what follows, a brief overview of what Moringa has been shown to do. As amazing as it may seem, no one suspected that cancer, diabetes and heart disease could be affected nutritionally as well. We should also understand that there are no therapeutic regimens that work for everyone and that the suggestions in this book do not take the place of a highly qualified medical practitioner. Now it is time to look at the physiological changes that are attributed to this hardy tree.

As was mentioned previously, Lowell Fuglie, of Dakar, is one of the foremost researchers on Moringa in the world. He believes that this plant, called "Nebeday" in Senegal, is the answer to malnutrition in Africa. Malnutrition kills up to twenty percent of the infants in Africa's poorest countries and under nutrition kills seven million worldwide.[505] [506] "Malnutrition is frequently characterized by this kind of restricted diet wherein a child consumes the same weaning pap every day. In this context, Moringa is a very simple and readily available solution to the problem of malnutrition. The edible leaves of the *Moringa oleifera* tree are already an occasional food source throughout West Africa and other regions of the tropics and sub-tropics. As a source of vitamin A and iron they are among the best of tropical legumes. In addition, Moringa leaves offer very significant quantities of vitamin C, B-complex, vitamins, calcium, protein, potassium, magnesium, selenium, zinc and a good balance of all the essential amino acids."[507] In addition to the vitamins, minerals and proteins mentioned by Fuglie, Moringa's nutrient list also include phytonutrients such as catechol tannins, gallic tannins, steroids, polysaccharides, triterpenoids, flavonoids, saponins,

---

[505] Population Reference Bureau, 1997. Population mondiale. Washington, D.C.
[506] Fuglie L J. Combating Malnutrition with Moringa. Development Potential for Moringa Products. *Church World Service*. Oct 29 to Nov 2, 2001.
[507] Fuglie L J. Combating Malnutrition with Moringa. Development Potential for Moringa Products. *Church World Service*. Oct 29 to Nov 2, 2001.

anthraquinones, alkaloids and reducing sugars just to name a few.[508]

Aside from this monumental finding that could affect millions of people around the world, Fuglie maintains that Moringa is also a remedy of choice for the common cold, infection, bronchitis, syphilis, dental cavities, earache, headache, toothaches, typhoid, warts, parasitic worms, throat infection, fever, epilepsy, prostate disorders.[509] It acts as a milk enhancer for lactating mothers, an aphrodisiac, antiseptic, and an astringent. Furthermore he goes on to state that it enhances prostate function, prevents prostate cancer, prevents anemia, and protects heart function by acting as a blood pressure lowering agent. He has found that it is good for digestive disorders, fertility, improving immune system function and almost every inflammatory disease known to man.[510]

Although much of Fuglie's findings have not been the result of double blind, controlled placebo studies, Fahey's comment (2005) assigns a degree of credibility to Moringa. "In fact, the nutritional properties of Moringa are now so well known that there seems to be little doubt of the substantial health benefit to be realized by consumption of Moringa leaf powder in situations where starvation is imminent. Nonetheless, the outcomes of well controlled and well documented clinical studies are still clearly of great value."[511]

---

[508] Bennet R N, Mellon F A, Foidl N, Pratt J H, DuPont M S, Perkins L, Kroon P A. Profiling glucosinolates and phenolics in vegetative and reproductive tissues of the multi-purpose trees Moringa oleifera L. (Horseradish tree) and Moringa stenopetala L. *J Agricultural and Food Chemistry*. 2003;51:p.3546-3553.
[509] Fuglie L J. *The Miracle Tree: Moringa oleifera: Natural Nutrition for the Tropics*. Church World Service, Dakar. 1999:68pp.
[510] ibid
[511] Fahey J W. *Moringa oleifera*: a review of the medical evidence for its nutritional, therapeutic, and prophylactic properties. *Trees for Life Journal*. 2005;1(5) p. 1-13.

In fact, Fuglie's findings about the miracle tree's abilities are corroborated in Paliwal et al (2011).[512] Paliwal and the team of researchers have published three papers on Moringa in 2011 alone, and their findings demonstrate a broad spectrum of protective effects conferred by the 'horse radish tree'.[513] [514] In the Asian Journal of Biotechnology, Paliwal has outlined the important medicinal uses of Moringa to be: anti-inflammatory, antioxidant, anti-cholesterol, enhancing skin health, increasing energy, improving vision, normalizing blood pressure, anti-depressant, strengthening the immune system, anti-fungal, reduction of age lines and wrinkles, anti tumor, improving wound healing, improving digestion, anti-ulcer, detoxification, appetite suppression, and normalizing blood sugar.[515]

With the escalating health care costs and the escalating incidence of disease, the introduction of *Moringa oleifera* as part of your daily diet can only have benefits. Paliwal cites multiple researchers and their findings and the list of applications for Moringa to combat disease and infection continues. (See Table V)[516]

---

[512] Paliwal R, Sharma V, Pracheta V. A review on Horse Radiah Tree (Moringa oleifera): A Multipurpose Tree with High Economic and Commercial Importance. *Asian Journal of Biotechnology*. 2011;3(4):p.317-328.

[513] Paliwal R, Sharma V, Pracheta V, Sharma S. Elucidation of free radical scavenging and antioxidant activity of aequeous and hydro-ethanolic extracts of Moringa oleifera pods. *Res J Pharm Tech*. 2011a;4:p.566-571.

[514] Paliwal R, Sharma V, Pracheta V, Sharma S H. Hepatoprotective and antioxidant potential of Moringa oleifera pods against DMBA-Induced hepatocarcinogenesis in male mice. *J Drug Dev Res*. 2011c (In press)

[515] Paliwal R, Sharma V, Pracheta V. A review on Horse Radish Tree (Moringa oleifera): A Multipurpose Tree with High Economic and Commercial Importance. *Asian Journal of Biotechnology*. 2011;3(4):p.324.

[516] Paliwal R, Sharma V, Pracheta V. A review on Horse Radiah Tree (Moringa oleifera): A Multipurpose Tree with High Economic and Commercial Importance. *Asian Journal of Biotechnology*. 2011;3(4):p.317-328.

TABLE 5
DISORDERS AFFECTED BY MORINGA

Disorders	Researchers
Abdominal swelling, rheumatism	Anwar F, Latif S, Ashraf M, Gilani A H. *Moringa oleifera*: A food plant with multiple medicinal uses. *Phytother Res.* 2007;21:p.17-25.
Cancer, hematological disorders, hepatic and renal function	Mazumder U K, Gupta M, Chakrabarty S,Pal D K. Evaluation of hematological and hepatorenal functions of methanolic extract of *Moringa oleifera* Lam. root treated mice. *Indian J Exp Biol.* 1999;37(6):p.612-614.
Cardiac function	Limaye D A, Nimbkar A Y, Jain R, Ahmad M.(1995) Cardiovascular effects of the aqueous extract of *Moringa pterygosperma*. *Phytotherapy Research* 1995;9:p.37-40.
Degenerative diseases, inflammation, infectious diseases, cardiovascular, gastrointestinal, hematological and hepatorenal disorders	Paliwal R, Sharma V, Pracheta V. A review on Horse Radiah Tree (*Moringa oleifera*): A Multipurpose Tree with High Economic and Commercial Importance. *Asian Journal of Biotechnology.* 2011;3(4):p.317-328.
Liver disease	Rao K S, Misra S H. Anti-inflammatory and antihepatotoxic activities of the rats of Moringa pterygosperma. *Geaertn Ind J Pharma Sci.* 1998;60:p.12-16.
Skin, hair, body conditioner (benoil)	Ramachandran C, Peter K V, Gopalakrishnan P K. 1980, Drumstick (*Moringa*

	oleifera): A multipurpose Indian Vegetable. *Economic Botany*, 34 (3) p.276-283. Marcu M G. Miracle Tree. KOS Health Publications. La Canada, CA. 2005;172pp.
Venomous bites, inflammation	Ezeamuzie I C, Ambakederemo A W, Shode F O, Ekwebelm S C. Antiinflammatory effects of *Moringa oleifera* root extract. *Int J Pharmacog*. 1996;34(3):p.207-212.

Due to the health oriented nature of this book, I have not dealt with the 'drumstick tree' as a food source, inexpensive water purification resource or major economic boon, but these potential impacts should not be overlooked. Although you have been given lists upon lists of diseases, disorders, and maladies, the quality and volume of research on Moringa simply cries out to be noticed.

Current estimates are that one in three people will suffer from cancer in their lifetime and even more from heart disease.[517] [518] [519] More than three and a half million in North America are afflicted by allergies so intense that they miss time from work. More than 20,000,000 people suffer from asthma and six thousand people die every year Thousands more have been stricken with autoimmune diseases. One million three hundred thousand people were diagnosed with cancer in the year 2000. "If cancer rates follow current patterns, we anticipate a doubling from 1.3 million people in 2000 to 2.6 million people in 2050 diagnosed with cancer," said Holly Howe, executive director of the North American Association of Central

---

[517] Lane William, Baxter Susan. Immune Power. Garden City Park, New York. Avery Publishing Group. 1999; p 119.
[518] Simone C. Cancer & Nutrition. Garden City Park, New York. Avery Publishing Group. 1992; p3.
[519] http://www.cdc.gov/nchs/fastats/lcod.htm

Cancer Registries.[520] The incidence of cancer currently affects forty-four percent (44%) of all men and thirty-nine percent (39%) of all women. [521] "The lifetime risks of dying from cancer are now 24% for men, and 20% for women." [522] Remember from Table I, a population of 308,000,000 has yielded 392,000,000 diseases...so who's healthy?

The correlation between nutrition and many of the chronic diseases exists and one does not have to have a deficiency status to be affected, only a sub-optimal intake. This is perhaps the beginning of a new generation of medicine where we might find a blending of alternative medicine with allopathic values. *Moringa oleifera* is one of the best candidates to fill this niche. It is time to do all that we can to improve our immune system health, increase our resistance to disease and in doing so; affect our over-all state of health. Optimize your nutritional protocols to the best of your ability. The threats to your health will never stop.

---

[520] CNN.com/Health. Report finds U.S. cancer rates declining but number of cases expected to double in next 50 years. May 14, 2002. <http://www.cnn.com/2002/HEALTH/05/14/cancer.statistics/?related.
[521] Epstein, S S. The Stop Cancer Before It Starts Campaign. Chicago. The Cancer Prevention Coalition. 2003; p5.
[522] Epstein, S S. *The Stop Cancer Before It Starts Campaign*. Chicago. The Cancer Prevention Coalition. 2003; p6.

Bibliography

Aben A, Danckaerts M. Omega-3 and omega-6 fatty acids in the treatment of children and adolescents with ADHD. *Tijdschr Psychiatr*.2010;52(2):p.89-97.

Abrams B, Duncan D, Hertz-Piccioto I. A prospective study ofdietary intake and acquired immune deficiency syndrome in HIV-sero-positive homosexual men. *J Acquired Immune Deficiency Syndrome*. 1993;8:p.949-958.

Adams P F, Martinez M E, Vickerie J L. *Summary Health Statistics for the U.S. Population: National Health Interview Survey*, 2009. National Center for Health Statistics. Vital Health Stat 10(248). 2010.

Agency for Toxic Substances and Disease Registry (ATSDR). *Toxilogical Profile for DDT, DDE, and DDD*. Update. Atlanta, GA. U.S. Department of Health and Human Services, Public Health Service. 2002.

Agrawal B, Mehta A. Antiasthmatic activity of Moringa oleifera Lam: A clinical study. *Indian J Pharma*. 2008;40(1):p.28-31.

Akhtar AH, Ahmad K U(1995) Anti-ulcerogenic evaluation of the methanolic extracts of some indigenous medicinal plants of Pakistan in aspirin-ulcerated rats. *J Ethnopharmacology* 1995;46:p.1-6.

Agnusdei D, Crepaldi G, Isaia G, et al. A double blind, placebo-controlled trial of ipriflavone for prevention of postmenopausal spinal bone loss. *Calcif Tissue Int*. 1997;61:p.142-147.

Allsopp R C, Harley C B, Evidence for a critical telomere length in senescent human fibroblasts. *Experimental Cell Res*. 1995;219:p.130-136.

Anderson D M W, Bell D C, et al. The gum exudates from *Chloroxylon swietenia, Sclerocarya caffra, Azadirachta indica* and *Moringa oleifera. Phytochemistry*. 1986;25(1):p.247-249.

Anderson H A, Lilis R, Selikoff I J et al. "Unanticipated prevelance of symptoms among dairy farmers in Michigan and Wisconsin." Environ Health Perspect. 1978; 23: p217-226.

Anderson R A, Cheng N, Bryden N A, Polansky M M, et al. Beneficial effects of chromium for people with diabetes. *Diabetes*. 1997; 46:p1786–1791.

Andersson S A. *Pain control by sensory stimulation*. In: Bonica J J ed. Advances in pain research and therapy. Vol 3. New York. Raven ress. 1979; p561-585.

Andrew P J, Myer B. Enzymatic function of nitric oxide synthases. *Cardiovascular Research*. 1999;43(3):p.521-531.

Angerer P, von Schacky C. n-3 polyunsaturated fatty acids and the cardiovascular system. *Curr Opin Lipidol*. 2000;11(1):p.57-63.

Anhwange B A, Ajibola V O, Oniye S J. Chemical studies of the seeds of *Moringa oleifera*(Lam) and Detarium microcarpum (Guill and Sperr). *J Biological Sci*. 2004;4:p.711-715.

Anwar F, Bhanger M I. Analytical characterization of *Moringa oleifera* seed oil grown in temperate regions of Pakistan. *J Agricultural and Food Chemistry* 2003;51:p.6558-6563.

Anwar F, Latif S, Ashraf M, Gilani A H. *Moringa oleifera*: A food plant with multiple medicinal uses. *Phytother Res*. 2007;21:p.17-25.

Appel L J, Miller E R , Seidler A J, et al. Does supplementation of diet with 'fish oil' reduce blood pressure? A meta-analysis of controlled clinical trials. *Arch Intern Med*. 1993;153:p.1429-1438.

Ashok K, Pari, L. Antioxidant action of *Moringa oleifera* Lam. (drumstick) against antitubercular drugs induced lipid peroxidation in rats. J Med Food. 2003; Fall; 6 (3):p.255-9.

Asres K. The major constituents of the acetone fraction of Ethiopian *Moringa stenopetala* leaves. *Mansoura Journal of Pharmacological Science*. 1995;11(1):p.55-64.
Austin M. *Acupuncture therapy*. New York. ASI Publishers. 1972.

Babu S C. Rural nutrition interventions with indigenous plant foods: a case study of vitamin deficiency in Malawi. International Food Policy Research Institute, Washington, DC. *Biotechnology, Agronomy Soc. Environ*. 2000 ;4(3):p.169-179.

Badgett B L. Part I. The mustard oil glucoside from *Moringa oleifera* seed. Rice University PhD Thesis (student of Martin G. Ettlinger), Houston, TX, USA. 1964.

Bahadori B, Uitz E, Thonhofer R, et al. omega-3 fatty acids infusions as adjuvant therapy in rheumatoid arthritis. *JPEN J Parenter Enteral Nutr*. 2010;34(2):p.151-5.

Balch P. *Prescription for Herbal Healing*. New York. Avery Publishing Group. 2002.

Balch J, Balch P. *Prescription for Nutritional Healing*. New York. Avery Publishing Group. 2000.

Balk E M, Lichtenstein A H, Chung M et al. Effects of omega-3 fatty acids on serum markers of cardiovascular disease risk: A systematic review. *Atherosclerosis*. 2006;189(1):p.19-30.

Barminas J T, Charles M, Emmanuel D. Mineral composition of non-conventional leafy vegetables. *Plant Foods for Human Nutrition* Dordrecht 1998;53(1):p.29-36.

Baron R. Effects of negative ions on cognitive performance. *Journal of Applied Psychology*. 1987; 72: p131-137.

Barrett R, Kuzawa W, McDade T, Armelagos G J. "Emerging and Re-Emerging Infectious Diseases: The Third Epidemiological Transition". *Annu Rev Anthropol*. 1998; (27): p.247-71.

Beach Rex. *Modern Miracle Men*. Washington. United States Government Printing Office Document No. 264. 1941.

Benhamou P Y, Mullen Y, Clare-Salzer M, et al. Essential fatty acid deficiency prevents autoimmune diabetes in non-obese diabetic mice through a positive impact on antigen-presenting cells and Th2 lymphocytes. *Pancreas*. 1995;11(1):p.26-37.

Bennett R N, Mellon F A, Foidl N, Pratt J H, DuPont M S, Perkins L, Kroon P A. Profiling glucosinolates and phenolics in vegetative and reproductive tissues of the multi-purpose trees *Moringa oleifera* L. (Horseradish tree) and *Moringa stenopetala* L. *J Agricultural and Food Chemistry*. 2003;51: p.3546-3553.

Berbert A A, Kondo C R, Almendra C L et al. Supplementation of fish oil and olive oil in patients with rheumatoid arthritis. *Nutrition*. 2005;21:p.131-136.

Berger M R, Habs M, Jahn S A, Schmahl S. Toxicological assessment of seeds from *Moringa oleifera* and *Moringa stenopetala*, two highly efficient primary coagulants for domestic water treatment of tropical raw waters. *East African Medical Journal* 1984;61:p.712-716.

Berkow R, Talbott J, Editors. *The Merck Manual Thirteenth Edition*. Rahway. Merck Sharpe and Dohme Research Laboratories. 1977. p241-243.

Bezerra A M E, Momente V G, Medeiros F S. Germinação de sementes e desenvolvimento de plântulas de moringa (*Moringa oleifera* Lam.) em função do peso da semente e do tipo de substrato. Hortic Bras. 2004;22:p.295-9.

Bharali R, Tabassum J, Azad M R H. Chemomodulatory effect of *Moringa oleifera*, Lam, on hepatic carcinogen metabolizing enzymes, antioxidant parameters and skin papillomagenesis in mice. *Asian Pacific Journal of Cancer Prevention* 2003;4:p.131-139.

Blackburn et al. Telomeres and telomerase: The path from maize, *Tetrahymena* and yeast to human cancer and aging. *Nature Medicine*. 2006;12:p.1133-1138.

Boelsma E, Hendriks HF. Roza L. Nutritional skin care: health effects of micronutrients and fatty acids. *Am J Clin Nutr*. 2001;73(5):p.853-864.

Brostow D P, Odegaard A O, Koh W P, Duval S, Gross M D, Yuan J M, Pereira M A. Omega-3 fatty acids and incident type 2 diabetes: the Singapore Chinese Health Study, 2011;94(2):p.520-526.

Brunader R, Shelton D K. Radiologic Bone Assessment in the Evaluation of Osteoporosis. *Am Fam Physician*. 2002; p1357-1364.

Buckalew L W, Rizzoto A. Subjective Response to Negative Air Ion Exposure. Journal of Aviation, *Space and Environmental Medicine*. August 1982; p822-823.

Burgess J, Stevens L, Zhang W, Peck L. Long-chain polyunsaturated fatty acids in children with attention-deficit hyperactivity disorder. *Am J Clin Nutr*. 2000;71(suppl):p.327S-330S.

Caceres A, O Cabrera, O Morales, P Mollinedo, P Mendia. Pharmacological properties of *Moringa oleifera*. 1: Preliminary screening for antimicrobial activity. *J Ethnopharmacology* 1991;33:p.213-216.

Caceres A, Lopez S. Pharmacological properties of *Moringa oleifera*: 3. Effect of seed extracts in the treatment of experimental pyodermia. *Fitoterapia*. 1991. 62(5):p.449-450.

Caceres A, Saravia A, Rizzo S, Zabala L, Leon E D, Nave F. Pharmacological properties of *Moringa oleifera*. 2: Screening for antispasmodic, anti-inflammatory and diuretic activity. *J Ethnopharmacol*. 1992;36:p.233-237.

Calo L, Bianconi L, Colivicchi F et al. N-3 Fatty acids for the prevention of atrial fibrillation after coronary artery bypass surgery: a randomized, controlled trial. *J Am Coll Cardiol.* 2005;45:p.1723-1728.

Castaneda F, Burse A, Boland W, Kinne R K H. Thioglycosides as inhibitors of hSGLT1 and hSGLT2: Potential therapeutic agents for the control of hyperglycemia in diabetes. *Int J Med Sci* 2007;4:p.131-139.

Centers for Disease Control and Prevention. *Cytomegalovirus.* National Center for Infectious Diseases. October 26, 2002. <http://www.cdc.gov/ncidod/diseases/cmv.htm.

Challem Jack. *10 Reasons to take supplements.* Aloha, Ore. The Nutrition Reporter. October/November 1996; p7-9.

Chandra RK. *Effect of Vitamin and Trace Element Supplementation on Immune Response in Elderly Subjects.* Lancet. 1992. 340:1124-1127.

Chandra RK. *Nutrition and the Immune System; an introduction.* Am J Clin Nutr. 1997b. 66:460S-463S.

Chandra R K. Nutrition, immunity and infection: present knowledge and future directions. Lancet. 1983; 1: p.688-691.

Chapel Helen. *Essentials of Clinical Immunology, 4th Edition.* Oxford. Blackwell Science. 1999. p21.

Chawla S, Saxena A, et al. In-vitro availability of iron in various green leafy vegetables. *Journal of the Science of Food and Agriculture* 1988;46(1): 125-128.

Cherry Laurence. *On the real benefits of Eustress: An Interview with Hans Selye.* Psychology Today. March 1978. p60.
Chopra, D. Ageless Body, Timeless Mind. New York. Harmony Books. 1993.

Chuang P H, Lee C W, Chou J Y, Murugan M, Shieh B J, Chen H M. Anti-fungal activity of crude extracts and essential oil of *Moringa oleifera* Lam. *Bioresource Technology.* 2007;Jan;98(1):p.232-236.

Chumark P, Khunawat P, Sanvarinda Y, Phornchirasilp S, Morales N P, Phivthong-ngam L, Ratanachamnong P, Srisawat S, Pongrapeeporn K-S. The *in vitro* and *ex vivo* antioxidant properties, hypolipidaemic and antiatherosclerotic activities of water extract of *Moringa oleifera* Lam. leaves. *J Ethnopharmacology.* 2008; 116:p.439-446.

CNN.com/Health. *Report finds U.S. cancer rates declining but number of cases expected to double in next 50 years.* May 14, 2002. <http://www.cnn.com/2002/HEALTH/05/14/cancer.statistics/?related.

Cole G M. Omega-3 fatty acids and dementia. *Prostaglandins Leukot Essent Fatty Acids.* 2009; 81(2-3):p.213-21.

Conquer J A, Tierney M C, Zecevic J, Bettger W J, Fisher R H. Fatty acid analysis of blood plasma of patients with Alzheimer's disease other types of dementia and cognitive impairment. *Lipids.* (2000);35:1301-1312.

Costa-Lotufo LV, Khan M T H, Ather A, Wilke D V, Jimenez P C, Pessoa C, MEA de Moraes MO de Moraes (2005) Studies of the anticancer potential of plants used in Bangladeshi folk medicine. *J Ethnopharmacology* 2005;99: p.21-30.

Cousens G. There Is a Cure for Diabetes: The Tree of Life 21-Day+ Program. North Atlantic Books, Berkeley, CA. 2008;446pp.

Crinnion W J. Environmental Medicine, Part 1: The Human Burden of Environmental Toxins and Their Common Health Effects. *Altern Med Rev.* 2000; 5(1):p52-63.

Curtis L T, Patel K. Nutritional and environmental approaches to preventing and treating autism and attention deficit hyperactivity disorder (ADHD): a review. *J Altern Complement Med.* 2008; 2008;14(1):p.79-85.

Curtis C L, Rees S G, Little C B, et al. Pathologic indicators of degradation and inflammation in human osteoarthritic cartilage are abrogated by exposure to n-3 fatty acids. *Arthritis Rheum.* 2002;46(6):p.1544-1553.

D'Souza J, Kulkarni A R. Comparative studies on nutritive values of tender foliage of seedlings and mature plants of *Moringa oleifera* Lam. *Journal of Economic and Taxonomic Botany* 1993;17(2):p.479-485.

Dahot M U. Antimicrobial activity of small protein of *Moringa oleifera* leaves. *Journal of the Islamic Academy of Sciences* 1998;11(1): 6 pp.

Dahot M U, Ali S A, et al. (1985) Proteolytic enzymes of *Moringa oleifera* seeds. *Journal of Pharmacy* 1985;6(1-2):p.1-10.

Dahot M U, Memon A R. Nutritive significance of oil extracted from *Moringa oleifera* seeds. *Journal of Pharmacy of the University of Karachi* 1985;3(2):p.75-80.

Dahot M U, Memon A R. Properties of *Moringa oleifera* seed lipase. *Pakistan Journal of Scientific and Industrial Research* 1987;30(11):p.832-835.

Daniel C R, McCullough M L, Patel R C, Jacobs E J, Flanders W D, Thun M J, Calle E E. Dietary intake of omega-6 and omega-3 fatty acids and risk of colorectal cancer in a prospective cohort of U.S. men and women. *Cancer Epidemiol Biomarkers Prev.* 2009;18(2):p.516-525.

Das B R, Kurup P A, Narasimha Rao P L. Antibiotic principle from *Moringa pterygosperma*. *Naturwissenschaften* 1954;41:p.66.

Das B R, Kurup P A, Narasimha Rao P L. Antibiotic principle from *Moringa pterygosperma*. Part VII. Anti-bacterial activity and chemical structure of compounds related to pterygospermin. *Indian J Med Res.* 1957;45:p.191-196

Das B R, Kurup P A, Narasimha Rao P L, Ramaswamy A S. Antibiotic principle from *Moringa pterygosperma*. Part VIII. Some pharmacological properties and in vivo action of pterygospermin and related compounds. *Indian J Med Res.* 1957;45:p.197-206.

Daub J R, Sandok B A, et al. *Medical Neurosciences: An Approach to Anatomy, Pathology, and Physiology by Systems and Levels.* Little Brown and Company. Boston. 1979; p382-383.

Dayrit F M, Alcantar A D, Villasenor I M. Studies on *Moringa oleifera* seeds, Part I: The antibiotic compound and its deactivation in aqueous solution. *Philippine Journal of Science.* 1990;119:p.23-32.

Dawson-Hughes B et al. *Effect of calcium and vitamin supplementation on bone density in men and women 65 years of age and older.* New Engl J Med. 1997; 337:670-676.

Delaveau P, et al. Oils of *Moringa oleifera* and Moringa drouhardii. *Plantes Médicinales et Phytothérapie.* 1980;14(10):p.29-33.

Delisle H, Bakari S, et al. Provitamin A content of traditional green leaves from Niger. *Cahiers Agricultures* 1997;6(6):p,553-560 de Lorgeril M, Salen P, Martin J L, et al. Mediterranean diet, traditional risk factors, and the rate of cardiovascular complications after myocardial infarction: final report of the Lyon Diet Heart Study. *Circulation*. 1999;99:p.779–785.

Dhar B, Gupta O P. Nutritional value of Shigru (*Moringa oleifera* Lam). *B M E B R*. 1982;3(2-4):p.280-288.

Dickinson A, Ed. *The Benefits of Nutritional Supplements*. Washington. Council For Responsible Nutrition. 1998.

Donli P, Dauda, H. Evaluation of aqueous Moringa seed extract as a seed treatment biofungicide for groundnuts. *Pest Manag Sci*. 2003; Sep; 59 (9):p.1060-1062.

Drinking Water, Pollution Prevention and Public Health: A matrix for Disease Prevention and Environmental Protection. United States Environmental Protection Agency, Office of Pollution, Prevention and Toxics. EPA Document 742-F-97-004. Washington. February 1997.

Drinking Water Standards. United States Environmental Protection Agency. <http://www.epa.gov/OGWDW/standards.html.

Duke J A. Moringaceae: Horseradish-tree, benzolive-tree, drumstick-tree, sohnja, moringa, murunga-kai, malunggay, p. 19-28. In: M. Benge (ed.) *Moringa: A multipurpose vegetable and tree that purifies water*. Sci. & Technol./ For., Environ., & Natural Resources Agro-Forestation Tech. Ser. 27. US AID, Washington, D.C. 1987.

Eilert U. Antibiotic principles of seeds of *Moringa oleifera*. *Indian Medical Journal*. 1978;38(235):p.1013-1016.

Eilert U, Wolters B, Nahrstedt A. The antibiotic principle of seeds of *Moringa oleifera* and *Moringa stenopetala*. *Planta Medica* 1981;42: p.55-61.

Epstein S. *The Stop Cancer Before It Starts Campaign*. Chicago. The Cancer Prevention Coalition. February 2003.

Ezeamuzie I C, Ambakederemo A W, Shode F O, Ekwebelm S C. Antiinflammatory effects of *Moringa oleifera* root extract. *Int J Pharmacog*. 1996;34(3):p.207-212.

Fahey J W. *Moringa oleifera*: a review of the medical evidence for its nutritional, therapeutic, and prophylactic properties. *Trees for Life Journal*. 2005;1(5) p. 1-13.

Fahey J W, Haristoy X, Dolan P M, Kensler T W, Scholtus I, Stephenson K K, Talalay P, Lozniewski A. Sulforaphane inhibits extracellular, intracellular, and antibiotic-resistant strains of *Helicobacter pylori* and prevents benzo[*a*]pyrene-induced stomach tumors. *Proceedings of the National Academy of Sciences USA* 2002;99:p.7610-7615.

Fahey J W, Dinkova-Kostova A T, Talalay P. *The "Prochaska" microtiter plate bioassay for inducers of NQO1*. Chapter 14 in Methods in Enzymology, Vol. 382, Part B, 2004;p. 243-258 (Eds.) H. Sies & L. Packer, Elsevier Science, San Diego, CA. 2004.

Fahey J W, Zalcmann A T, Talalay P. The chemical diversity and distribution of glucosinolates and isothiocyanates among plants. *Phytochemistry*. 2001;56(1):p.5-51.

Faizi S, et al. Novel hypotensive agents, niazimin A, niazimin B, niazicin A and niazicin B from *Moringa oleifera*: Isolation of first naturally occurring carbamates. *Journal of the Chemical Society Perkin Transactions I:* 1994;p.3035-3040.

Faizi S, BS Siddiqui, et al. Isolation and structure elucidation of novel hypotensive agents, niazinin A, niazinin B, niazimicin and niaziminin A plus B from *Moringa oleifera*: The first naturally occurring thiocarbamates. *Journal of the Chemical Society Perkin Transactions*. 1992;I(23):p.3237-3241.

Faizi S, Siddiqui B S, Saleem R, Aftab K, Shaheen F, Gilani A H. Bioactive Compounds from the leaves and pods of *Moringa oleifera*. *New Trends in Natural Products Chemistry* 1998;p.175-183.

Faizi S, Siddiqui B S, Saleem R, Aftab K, Shaheen F, Gilani A H. Hypotensive constituents from the pods of *Moringa oleifera*. *Planta Medica* 1998;64:p.225-228.

Faizi S, Siddiqui B S, Saleem R, Aftab K, Shaheen F, Gilani A H. Fully acetylated carbamate and hypotensive thiocarbamate glycosides from *Moringa oleifera*. *Phytochemistry* 1995;38:p.957-963.

Faizi S, Siddiqui B S, Saleem R, Aftab K, Shaheen F, Gilani A H. Isolation and structure elucidation of new nitrile and mustard oil glycosides from *Moringa oleifera* and their effect on blood pressure. *Journal of Natural Products* 1994;57:p.1256-1261.

Fisher H W. Acute Low Back Pain Treated by Spinal Manipulation and Electronic Acupuncture. *J Manipulative Physiol Ther*. 1992; 15: p199-202.

Fisher, H W. *Wisdom of the Woods: Herbal Remedies*. Wood Publishing. Toronto. 2002; p3.

Fletcher D J. Warming up to Far-Infrared. *Alternative Medicine Magazine*. Jan 2001: 39.

Foidl N, Paull R. *Moringa oleifera* In: *The Encyclopedia of Fruit and Nuts*, Janick j and Paull R E (Eds). CABI, Oxfordshire, UK. 2008;p.509-512.

Fotuhi M, Mohassel P, Yaffe K. Fish consumption, long-chain omega-3 fatty acids and risk of cognitive decline or Alzheimer disease: a complex association. *Nat Clin Pract Neurol*. 2009;5(3):p.140-152.

Frank, Michael ed. *Overview of the Immune System, Vol 1 Samter's Immunologic Disease, 5th Ed*. New York. Little Brown and Co.1995.

Frawley D. *Ayurvedic Healing*. Salt Lake City. Morson Publishing. 1990.

Freiberger C E, Vanderjagt D J, et al. Nutrient content of the edible leaves of seven wild plants from Niger. *Plant Foods for Human Nutrition* 1998;53(1): 57-69.

Friel J P, ed. *Dorland's Illustrated Medical Dictionary*. Twenty-fifth Edition. W.B. Saunders. Philadelphia. 1974.

Fuglie L J. *New Uses of Moringa Studied in Nicaragua*. ECHO Development Notes #68, June, 2000.

Fuglie L J. *The Miracle Tree: Moringa oleifera: Natural Nutrition for the Tropics*. Church World Service, Dakar. 1999:68pp.

Fuglie L J. Combating Malnutrition with Moringa. Development Potential for Moringa Products. *Church World Service*. Oct 29 to Nov 2, 2001.

Galan M V, Kishan A A, Silverman A A. Oral broccoli sprouts for the treatment of Helicobacter pylori infection: A preliminary report. *Dig Dis Sci*;2004;49(7-8):p.1088-1090.

Galarraga B, Ho M, Youssef H M, et al. Cod liver oil (n-3 fatty acids) as an non-steroidal anti-inflammatory drug sparing agent in rheumatoid arthritis. *Rheumatology* (Oxford) 2008;47(5):p.665-669.

Galli C, Risé P. Fish consumption, omega 3 fatty acids and cardiovascular disease. The science and the clinical trials. *Nutr Health.* 2009;20(1):11-20.

Ganguly R, Hazra R, Ray K, Guha D. Effect of *Moringa oleifera* in experimental model of Alzheimer's disease: Role of antioxidants. *Ann Neurosci.* 2005;12:p.36-9.

Ganguly R, Guha D. Protective role of an Indian herb, *Moringa oleifera* in memory impairment by high altitude hypoxic exposure: Possible role of monoamines. *Biogenic Amines.* 2006;20:p.121-33.

Gassenschmidt U, Jany K D, Tauscher B, Niebergall H. Isolation and characterization of a flocculating protein from *Moringa oleifera* Lam. *Biochimica Biophysica Acta.* 1995;1243:p.477-481.

Geervani P, Devi A. Influence of protein and fat on the utilisation of carotene from drumstick (*Moringa oleifera*) leaves. *Indian J Med Res.* 1981;74:p.548-553.

Ghasi S, Nwobodo E, Ofili J. Hypocholesterolemic effects of crude extract of leaf of *Moringa oleifera* Lam. in high-fat diet fed wistar rats. *J Ethnopharmacol.* 2000; Jan;69 (1):p.21-5.

Ghebremichael K A, Gunaratna K R, Henriksson H, Brumer H, Dalhammar G. A simple purification and activity assay of the coagulant protein from *Moringa oleifera* seed. Water Research. 2005;39:p.2338-2344.

Gilani A H, Aftab K, Suria A, Siddiqui S, Saleem R, Siddiqui B S, Faizi S. Pharmacological studies on hypotensive and spasmolytic activities of pure compounds from *Moringa oleifera. Phytotherapy Research* 1994;8(2):p.87-91.

Girija V, Sharada D, Pushpamma P. (Bioavailability of thiamine, riboflavin and niacin from commonly consumed green leafy vegetables in the rural areas of Andhra Pradesh in India. *Intl J Vitamin & Nutrition Research.* 1982;52:p.9-13.

Gokce N. L-Argenine and hypertension. *J Nutrition.* 2004;134(10 Suppl):p.2807S-2811S.

Goldberg R J, Katz J. A meta-analysis of the analgesic effects of omega-3 polyunsaturated fatty acid supplementation for inflammatory joint pain. *Pain.* 2007; May 29L1-2):p.210-223.

Gopalakrishna K S, Kurup P A Narashimha Rao P L. Antibiotic principles from *Moringa pterygosperma*. Part III. Action of pterygospermin on germination of seeds and filamentous fungi. *Indian J Med Res* 1954;42:p.97-99.

Grant G, More L J, McKenzie N H, Dorward P M, Stewart J C, Telek L, Pusztai A. Nutritional and haemagglutination properties of several tropical seeds. *J Agricultural Science*. 1995;124(3):p.437-445.

Guevara A P, Vargas C, Sakurai H, Fujiwara Y, Hashimoto K, Maoka T, Kozuka M, Ito Y, Tokuda H, Nishino H. An antitumor promoter from *Moringa oleifera* Lam. *Mutation Research* 1999;440:p.181-188.

Gunderson E L. *FDA Total Diet Survey, April 1982-April 1986, Dietary intakes of pesticides, selected elements and other chemicals.* Food and Drug Administration, Division of Contaminants Chemistry. Washington, DC 20204.

Gupta M, UK Mazumder U K, et al. CNS activities of methanolic extract of *Moringa oleifera* root in mice. *Fitoterapia*. 1999;70(3): 244-250.

Gupta M, UK Mazumder U K, et al. Anti-epileptic and anti-cancer activity of some indigenous plants. *Indian Journal of Physiology and Allied Sciences* 1997;51(2):p.53-56.

Guyton A C. *Textbook of Medical Physiology.* Second Edition. W.B. Saunders. Philadelphia. 1961. p64.

Haas, Elson M. *Staying Healthy With Nutrition: The Complete Guide to Diet and Nutritional Medicine.* Berkeley, California. Celestial Arts. 1992. p905-907.

Hagen K B, Byfuglien MG, Falzon L, Olsen SU, Smedslund G. Dietary interventions for rheumatoid arthritis. *Cochrane Database Syst Rev.* 2009; Jan 21;(1):CD006400.

Hameed-Un-Nisa L, Shehnaz D, Faizi S. (1998) Measurement of sympatholytic activity of *Moringa oleifera. New Trends in Natural Products Chemistry* [6th International Symposium on Natural Products Chemistry] Harwood Amsterdam. 1998;p.269-277.

Hartwell J L. Plants used against cancer: a survey. *Lloydia* 1971;p.30-34.

Haristoy X, Fahey J W, Scholtus I, Lozniewski A. Evaluation of antimicrobial effect of several isothiocyanates on *Helicobacter pylori*. *Planta Medica*. 2005;71: 326-330.

Haschek W M, Rousseaux C G. *Handbook of Toxicologic Pathology*. San Diego. Academic Press. 1991.

Hauser S L, Doolittle T H, Lopez-Bresnahan M, Shahani B, Schoenfeld D, Shih V E, Grodon J, Lehrich J R. An antispasticity effect of threonine in multiple sclerosis. *Arch Neurol*. 1992;49(9):p.923-926.

Hirsch, A. *Preliminary document on the nutritional value of leaves and pods of Moringa oleifera*. UCLA, Department of Botany. 2004.

Holman R T. The slow discovery of the importance of omega 3 essential fatty acids in human health. *J Nutr* 1998;128 (2 Suppl):p.427S–433S.

Hueser G. Diagnostic markers in clinical immunotoxicology and neurotoxicology. *J Occup Med Toxicol*. 1992; 1:p5-9.

Hoekman T. *Heavy metal toxicology*. <http://www.luminet.net/~wenonah/hydro/heavymet.htm.

Holst S. *Moringa: Nature's Medicine Cabinet*. Sierra Sunrise Publishing, Sherman Oaks, CA. 2000.128 pp.

Honda K, Inoue S. Sleep-enhancing effects of far infrared radiation in rats. *Int J Biometeorol*. 1988; 32: p32-34.

Howe GR, Benito E, Castelleto R et al. Dietary Intake of fiber and decreased risk of cancers of the colon and rectum: evidence from the combined analysis of 13 case control studies. *J Natl Cancer Inst*. 1992; 84:1887-1896.

Howe P R. Dietary fats and hypertension: focus on fish oil. *Ann N Y Acad Sci*. 1997;827:p.339–352.

Hukkeri V I, Nagathan C V, Karadi R V, Patil B S. Antipyretic and wound healing activities of *Moringa oleifera* Lam. In rats. *Indian J Pharmaceutical Sciences*. 2006;68(1):p.124-126.

Imai Kazue, Matsuyama Satoru et al. Natural cytotoxic activity of peripheral-blood lymphocytes and cancer incidence: an 11 year follow up study of a general population. *Lancet*. Vol 356 Issue 9244. November 2000; 1795-99.

Ionizing Radiation Exposure of the Population of the United States Report No. 93. National Council on Radiation Protection and Measurements. Bethesda MD. 1987.

Jabeen R, Shahid M, Jamil A, Ashraf M. Microscopic evaluation of the antimicrobial activity of seed extracts of *Moringa oleifera*. *Pak J Bot.* 2008;40:p.1349-58.

Jacquat C, Bertossa G. *Plants from the Markets of Thailand.* Editions Duang Kamol, Bangkok. 1990;p. 38.

Jadhav S L, Sharma S R, Pal S C, Kasture S B, Kasture V S. (2000) Chemistry and pharmacology of *Moringa oleifera* and *Moringa concanescens* Niro. *Indian Drugs* 2000;37(3):p.139-144.

Jahn S A. The traditional domestication of a multipurpose tree *Moringa stenopetala* (Bak.f.) Cuf. in the Ethiopian Rift Valley. 1991;20:p.244-247.

Jahn S A. On the introduction of a tropical multipurpose tree to China traditional and potential utilisation of *Moringa oleifera* Lamark. *Senckenbergiana Biologica* 1996;75(1-2):p.243-254.

Jahn S A, Musnad H A, Burgstaller H., Tree that purifies water: Cultivating multipurpose Moringaceae in the Sudan. *Unasylva* 1986;38(152):p.23-28.

Jansen J, Karges W, Rink L. Zinc and diabetes - clinical links and molecular mechanisms. *J Nut Biochem.* 2009;20(6):p.399-417.

Jayavardhanan K K, Suresh K, Panikkar K R, Vasudevan D M. Modulatory potency of drumstick lectin on the host defense system. *Journal of Experimental Clinical Cancer Research* 1994;13(3):p.205-209.

Jensen B, Bodeen D. *Visions of Health: Understanding Iridology.* New York. Avery Books. 1992.

Johnell O, Kanis J A. An estimate of the worldwide prevalence and disability associated with osteoporotic fractures. Osteoporos Int. 2006; 17:p.1726.

Johnson B C. Clinical perspectives on the health effects of *Moringa oleifera*: A promising adjunct for balanced nutrition and better health. KOS Health Publications August 2005: 1-5

Kanis J A. *WHO Technical Report*, University of Sheffield, UK. 2007:p.66

Kar A, Choundhary B, Bandyopadhyay N. Preliminary studies on the inorganic constituents of some indigenous hypoglycaemic herbs on oral glucose tolerance test. *J Ethnopharmacology*. 1999;64(2):p.179-184.

Kar A, Choundhary B, Bandyopadhyay N. Comparative evaluation of hypoglycaemic activity of some Indian medicinal plants in alloxan diabetic rats. *J Ethnopharmacol*. 2003;Jan; 84 (1):p.105-108.

Kastelan M, Kovacik K, Tarle, et al. Analysis of NK cell activity, lymphocyte reactivity to mitogens and serotest PSA and TPS values in patients with primary and disseminated prostate cancer, PIN and BPH. *Anticancer Res*. 1997;17:p.1671-1675.

Kjaer A, Malver O, El-Menshawi B, Reisch J. Isothiocyanates in myrosinase-treated seed extracts of *Moringa peregrina*. *Phytochemistry* 1979;18:p.1485-1487.

Klinghardt D. Metal Toxicity. *Explore*. 2000; Vol 10 (1).

Kopple J D, Swendseid M E. Evidence that histidine is an essential amino acid in nbormal and chronically uremic man. *J Clin Invest*. 1975;55(5):p.881-891.

Kotaka S. Effects of air ions on microorganisms and other biological materials. *CRC Critical Reviews in Microbiology*. 1978; 6: p109-149.

Kris-Etherton P, Eckel R H, Howard B V, St. Jeor S, Bazzare T L. AHA Science Advisory: Lyon Diet Heart Study. Benefits of a Mediterranean-style, National Cholesterol Education Program/American Heart Association Step I Dietary Pattern on Cardiovascular Disease. *Circulation*. 2001;103:p.1823.

Kremer J M. N-3 fatty acid supplements in rheumatoid arthritis. *Am J Clin Nutr*. 2000;(suppl 1)p.349S-351S.

Krishna Mohan I, Das UN. Prevention of chemically induced diabetes mellitus in experimental animals by polyunsaturated fatty acids. *Nutrition*. 2001; 17(2):126-151.

Kruger M, Horrobin D. Calcium metabolism, osteoporosis and essential fatty acids: a review. *Prog Lipid Res*.1997;36(2-3):131-151.

Kumar K, Goel A K. Frequently used ethno-medicinal plants of Bihar. *Journal of Economic and Taxonomic Botany*. 1999;23(2):p.645-649.

122 Moringa Oleifera

Kumar S, Gopal K (1999) Screening of plant species for inhibition of bacterial population of raw water. *J Environ Sci & Health: Part A Toxic Hazardous Substances and Environmental Engineering.* 1994;34(4):p.975-987.

Kumar N A, Pari I. Antioxidant action of *Moringa oleifera* Lam (drumstick) against antitubercular drug induced lipid peroxidation in rats. *J Medicinal Foods.* 2003;6(3):p.255-259.

Kurup P A, Narasimha Rao P L. Antibiotic principle from *Moringa pterygosperma.* Part IV. The effect of addition of vitamins and amino acids on the anti-bacterial activity of pterygospermin. *Indian J Med Res* 1954;42:p.101-107.

Kurup P A, Narasimha Rao P L. Antibiotic principle from *Moringa pterygosperma.* Part V. Effect of pterygospermin on the assimilation of glutamic acid by *Micrococcus pyogenes* var. *aureus. Indian J Med Res.* 1954;42:p.109-114.

Kurup P A, Narasimha Rao P L,Venkataraman R. Antibiotic principle from *Moringa pterygosperma.* Part VI. Mechanism of anti-bacterial action of pterygospermin inhibition of transaminase by pterygospermin. *Indian J Med Res.* 1954;42: 115-123.

Lane William, Baxter Susan. *Immune Power.* Garden City Park, New York. Avery Publishing Group. 1999.

Laza V, Olinic A, Ionut C. Action of the Negative Air Ions in Moderate Concentration on Laboratory Animals Treated with Zinc and Thyram. *CEJOEM.* 1998; Vol. 4. No. 1:p59-65.

Leoni V, Fabiani L, Marinelli G, et al. PCB and other organochlorine compounds in blood of women with or without miscarriage: a hypothesis of correlation. *Ecotoxicol Environ Saf.* 1989; 17.p1-11.

Leuck M, Kunz H. Synthesis of active principles from the leaves of *Moringa oleifera* using *S*-pent-4-enyl thioglycosides. *Carbohydrate Research* 1998;312(1-2):p.33-44.

Lewis K. "Multidrug resistance pumps in bacteria: variations on a theme". *Trends Biochem Sci.* 1994; 19(3): p.119-23.

Limaye D A, Nimbkar A Y, Jain R, Ahmad M.(1995) Cardiovascular effects of the aqueous extract of *Moringa pterygosperma. Phytotherapy Research* 1995;9:p.37-40.

Lipipun V, Kurokawa M, Suttisri R, Taweechotipatr P, Pramyothin P, Hattori M, Shiraki K. Efficacy of Thai medicinal plant extracts against herpes simplex virus type 1infection in vitro and in vivo. *Antivir Res*. 2003; Nov; 60(3):p.175-80.

Lockett C T, C. Calvert C C, et al. Energy and micronutrient composition of dietary and medicinal wild plants consumed during drought. Study of rural Fulani, Northeastern Nigeria. *Intl J Food Sciences and Nutrition*. 2000;51(3):p.195-208.

Maciocia G. *Tongue diagnosis in Chinese Medicine*. Vista, CA. Eastland Publishing. 1995.

Madsen M, Schlundt J, Omer E F. Effect of water coagulation by seeds of *Moringa oleifera* on bacterial concentrations. *J Trop Med & Hyg*. 1987;90:p.101-109.

Maggio M, Artoni A, Lauretani F, Borghi L, Nouvenne A, Valenti G, Ceda G P. The impact of omega-3 fatty acids on osteoporosis. *Curr Pharm Des*. 2009;15(36):p.4157-4164.

Mahajan S G, Banerjee A, Chauhan B F, Padh H, Nivsarkar M, Mehta A A. Inhibitory effect of n-butanol fraction of *Moringa oleifera* Lam. Seeds on ovalbumin-induced airway inflammation in a guinea pig model of asthma. *Int J Toxicol*. 2009;Nov-Dec;28(6):p.519-527.

Mahajan S G, Mali, R G, Mehta A A. Protective effect of ethanolic extract of seeds of *Moringa oleifera* Lam against inflammation associated with development of arthritis in rats. *J Immunotoxicol*. 2007;Jan;4(1):p.39-47.

Mahmood K T, Mugal T, Haq L U. *Moringa oleifera*: A natural gift- A review. *J Phar Sci* Res. 2010;2:p.775-781.

Majumdar K, Gupta M, Chakrobarty S, Pal DK. Evaluation of hematological and hepatorenal functions of methanolic extract of *Moringa oleifera* Lam. root treated mice. *Indian J Exp Biol* 1999;37:p.612-4.

Makkar H P S, Becker K. Nutrients and antiquality factors in different morphological parts of the *Moringa oleifera* tree. *J Agricultural Science* 1997;128(3):p.311-322.

Makkar H P S, Becker K. Nutritional value and antinutritional components of whole and ethanol extracted *Moringa oleifera* leaves. *Animal Feed Science and Technology* 1996;63(1-4):p.211-228.

124   Moringa Oleifera

Makkar H P S, Becker K. Nutrients and antiquality factors in different morphological parts of the *Moringa oleifera* tree. *J Agric Sci.* 1997;128:p.311-22.

Makonnen E, Hunde A, Damecha G. Hypoglycaemic effect of *Moringa stenopetala* aqueous extract in rabbits. *Phytotherapy Research* 1997;11:p.147-148.

Mandloi M, Chaudhari S, Folkard, G. Evaluation of natural coagulants for direct filtration. *Environ Technol.* 2004; Apr; 25 (4):p.481-9.

Mann F. *Acupuncture: the ancient Chinese art of healing and how it works scientifically.* New York. Vintage Books. 1973.
Marcu M G. *Miracle Tree.* KOS Health Publications, La Canada, CA. 2005;172 pp.

Maret W. Zinc and Diabetes. *Biometals.* 2005;18(4):p.293-294.
Martin F W, Ruberte R M, Meitzner L S. *Edible Leaves of the Tropics.* 3rd Ed. Educational Concerns for Hunger Organization, Inc., N. Ft. Meyers, FL. 1998;194 pp.

Mazumder U K, Gupta M, Chakrabarty S,Pal D K. Evaluation of hematological and hepatorenal functions of methanolic extract of *Moringa oleifera* Lam. root treated mice. *Indian J Exp Biol.* 1999;37(6):p.612-614.

McEntee W, Crook T. Glutamate: Its role in learning, memory and the aging brain. *Psychopharmacology.* 1993;111(4):p.391-401.

Mehta L K, Balaraman R, Amin A H, Bafna P A , Gulati O D. (2003) Effect of fruits of *Moringa oleifera* on the lipid profile of normal and hypocholesterolaemic rabbits. *J Ethnopharmacology* 2003;86:p.191-195.

Mekonnen Y. Effects of ethanol extract of *Moringa stenopetala* leaves on guinea-pig and mouse smooth muscle. *Phytotherapy Research* 1999;13:p.442-444.

Mekonnen Y, Drager B. Glucosinolates in *Moringa stenopetala. Planta Med.* 2003;69:p.380-382.

Mekonnen Y, Yardley V, Rock P, Croft S. In vitro antitrypanosomal activity of *Moringa stenopetala* leaves and roots. *Phytotherapy Research.* 1999;13:p.538-539.

Memon G M, Khatri L M. Isolation and spectroscopic studies of mono-palmitic, di-oleic triglyceride from seeds of *Moringa oleifera* Lam. *Pak J Sci & Ind Res*. 1987;30(5):p.393-395.

Memon G M, Memon S A, et al. Isolation and structure elucidation of moringyne: A new glycoside from seeds of *Moringa oleifera*. *Pakistan J Sci and Industrial Research* 1985;28(1):p.7-9.

Mohan M, Kaul N, Punekar A, Girnar R, Junnare P, Patil L. Nootropic activity of *Moringa oleifera* leaves. *J Nat Remedies*. 2005;5:p.59-62.

Mondal S, Chakraborty I, Pramanik M, Rout D, Islamm SS. Structural studies of an immunoenhancing polysaccharide isolated from mature pods (fruits) of *Moringa oleifera* (Sajina). Med Chem Res 2004;13:p.390-□400.

Monzon R B. Traditional medicine in the treatment of parasitic diseases in the Philippines. *Southeast Asian Journal of Tropical Medicine and Public Health*1995;26(3): 421-428.

Mori T A. Omega-3 fatty acids and blood pressure. *Cell Mol Biol (Nosiy-le-grand)*. 2010;56(1):p.83-92.

Morris M C, Sacks F, Rosner B. Does fish oil lower blood pressure? A meta-analysis of controlled trials. *Circulation*. 1993;88:p.523–533.

Morton J F. The horseradish tree, *Moringa pterygosperma* Moringaceae) – A boon to arid lands? *Economic Botany* 1991;45:p.318-333.

Mossa J S. A study on the crude antidiabetic drugs used in Arabian folk medicine. *Int J Crude Drug Research* 1985;23(3):p.137-145.

Muluvi G M, Sprent J I, Soranzo N, Provan J, Odee D, Folkard G, McNicol J W, Powell W. (1999) Amplified fragment length poly-morphism (AFLP) analysis of genetic variation in *Moringa oleifera* Lam. *Mol Eco*. 1999;8:p.463-470.

Murakami A, Kitazono Y, Jiwajinda S, Koshimizu K, Ohigashi H. Niaziminin, a thiocarbamate from the leaves of *Moringa oleifera*, holds a strict structural requirement for inhibition of tumor-promoter-induced Epstein-Barr virus activation. *Planta Medica* 1998;64: p.319-323.

Murphy SP, Rose D, Hudes M, Viteri FE. Demographic and economic factors associated with dietary quality for adults in 1987-1988

Nationwide Food Consumption Survey. *J Am Diet Assn*. 1992; 92:1352-1357.

Naidoo K K, Coopoosamy R M. Review on herbal remedies used by the 1860 South African Indian settlers. *African J Biotech*. 2011; 10 August:p. 8533-8538.

Nambiar V S, Seshadri S. Bioavailability trials of beta-carotene from fresh and dehydrated leaves of *Moringa oleifera* in a rat model. *Plant Foods for Human Nutrition*. 2001;56(1): 83-95.

Narasimha Rao P I, Kurup P A(1953) Pterygospermin – the antibiotic principle of *Moringa pterygosperma* Gaertn.. *Indian J Pharmacy*. 1953;15(12): p.315.

Nath D, Sethi N, et al. Survey on indigenous medicinal plants used for abortion in some districts of Uttar Pradesh. *Fitoterapia*. 1997;68(3);p.223-225.

Nath D, Sethi N, Singh R K, Jain A K. Commonly used Indian abortifacient plants with special reference to their teratologic effects in rats. *J Ethnopharmacology* 1992 ;36: 147-154.

National Cholesterol Education Program (NCEP) Expert Panel on Detection, Evaluation, and Treatment of High Blood Cholesterol in Adults (Adult Treatment Panel, III) (2002-12-17). "Third Report of the National Cholesterol Education Program (NCEP) Expert Panel on Detection, Evaluation, and Treatment of High Blood Cholesterol in Adults (Adult Treatment Panel III) final report." *Circulation*. 2002;106(25):p.3143-421.

National Council on Radiation Protection and Measurements. *Ionizing Radiation Exposure of the Population of the United States Report* No. 93. Bethesda MD. 1987.

Nature Works. *Body Detoxification, Toxins and the Immune System*. 2002. <http://immunedisorders.homestead.com/Detoxification.html.

Nature Works. *Immune Disorders*. 2002. <http://immunedisorders.homestead.com/booklet/html.
Nautiyal B P, Venkataraman K G. Moringa (Drumstick) – An ideal tree for social forestry: Growing conditions and uses – Part I. *MYFOREST*. 1987;23(1):p.53-58.

Nelson D L, Cox M M. Principles of Biochemistry (4 ed.), New York. W H Freeman. 2005;p684-685.

Neumann J, Winterton S, Foulds J, Smith R, Lu J. Toxic Nation: A Report on Pollution In Canadians. *Environmental Defence*. 2005.

Newcomer L M, King I B, Wicklund K G, Stanford J L. The association of fatty acids with prostate cancer risk. *Prostate*. 2001;47(4):p.262-268.

Njoku O U, Adikwu M U. Investigation on some physico-chemical antioxidant and toxicological properties of *Moringa oleifera* seed oil. *Acta Pharmaceutica Zagreb*. 1997;47(4):p.87-290.

Norris J, Yin X, Lamb M M, Barriga K, Seifert J, Hoffman M, Orton H D, Baron A E, Clare-Salzler M, Chase H P, Szabo N J, Erlich H, Eisenbarth G S, Rewers M. Omega-3 polyunsaturated fatty acid intake and island autoimmunity in children at increased risk for type I diabetes. *JAMA*. 2007;298(12):p.1420-1428.

Nwosu M O, Okafor J I. Preliminary studies of the antifungal activities of some medicinal plants against *Basidiobolus* and some other pathogenic fungi. *Mycoses*. 1995;38:p.191-195.

Obulesu O, Rao D M. Effect of plant extracts on Alzheimer's disease: An insight into therapeutic avenues. *J Neurosciences in Rural Practice*. 2011;2(1):p.56-61.

Oliveira J T A, Silveira S B, et al. Compositional and nutritional attributes of seeds from the multiple purpose tree *Moringa oleifera* Lamarck. *J Sci Food and Agriculture*. 1999;79(6):p.815-820.

Olsen A. Low technology water purification by bentonite clay and *Moringa oleifera* seed flocculation as performed in Sudanese villages. Effects on *Schistosoma mansoni* cercariae. *Water Research*. 1987;21(5): p.517-522.

Osiecki H, Meeke F, Smith J. *The Encyclopaedia of Clinical Nutrition-Volunme 1: The Nervous System*. BioConceps Publishing. Queensland. 2004.

Pal S K, Mukherjee P K, Saha K, Pal M, Saha B P. Antimicrobial action of the leaf extract of *Moringa oleifera* Lam. *Ancient Science of Life* 1995;14(3):p.197-199.

Pal S K, Mukherjee P K, Saha B P. Studies on the antiulcer activity of *Moringa oleifera* leaf extract on gastric ulcer models in rats. *Phytotherapy Research*. 1995;9:p.463-465.

Palada M C, Chang L C. Suggested cultivation practices for Moringa.
AVRDC Publication #03-545; 2003.
http://www.avrdc.org/LC/indigenous/moringa.pdf

Palada M C. Moringa (*Moringa oleifera* Lam.): A versatile tree crop
with horticultural potential in the subtropical United States. H*ort
Science* 1996;31:p.794-797.

Paliwal R, Sharma V, Pracheta V. A review on Horse Radiah Tree
(*Moringa oleifera*): A Multipurpose Tree with High Economic and
Commercial Importance. *Asian Journal of Biotechnology*.
2011;3(4):p.317-328.

Paliwal R, Sharma V, Pracheta V, Sharma S. Elucidation of free radical
scavenging and antioxidant activity of aequeous and hydro-ethanolic
extracts of *Moringa oleifera* pods. *Res J Pharm Tech*. 2011a;4:p.566-
571.

Paliwal R, Sharma V, Pracheta V, Sharma S, Yadav S, Sharma S H.
Antiephrotoxic effect of administration of *Moringa oleifera* Lam in
amelioration of dmba-induced renal carcinogenesis in swiss albino
mice. *Biol Med*. 2011b;p.25-35.

Paliwal R, Sharma V, Pracheta V, Sharma S H. Hepatoprotective and
antioxidant potential of *Moringa oleifera* pods against DMBA-induced
hepatocarcinogenesis in male mice. *Int J Drug Dev Res*. 2011c (in
press).

Panda D, Si S, Swain S, Kanungo S K, Gupta R. Preparation and
evaluation of gels from gum of *Moringa oleifera*. *Indian J
Pharmaceutical Sciences*. 2006;68(6):p.778-780.

Panda D, Choudhury N S K, Yedukondalu M, Si S, Gupta R.
Evaluation of gum of *Moringa oleifera* as a binder and release retardant
in tablet formation. *Indian J Pharmaceutical Sciences*.
2008;70(5):p.614-618.

Pankaja N, Prakash J.(1994) Availability of calcium from kilkeerai
(*Amaranthus tricolor*) and drumstick (*Moringa oleifera*) greens in
weanling rats. *Nahrung* 1994;38:p.199-203.

Pari L, Kumar N A. Hepatoprotective activity of *Moringa oleifera* on
antitubercular drug-induced liver damage in rats. *J Med Foods*.
2002;5(3): 171-177.

Prakash A O.Ovarian response to aqueous extract of *Moringa oleifera*
during early pregnancy in rats. *Fitoterapia* 1988;59(2): 89-96.

Prakash A O, Pathak S, Shukla S, Mathur R. (1987) Uterine histoarchitecture during pre and post-implantation periods of rats treated with aqueous extract of *Moringa oleifera* Lam. *Acta Europaea Fertilitatis* 1987;18: p.129-135.

Prasad R, Lawania R D, Manvi, Gupta R. Role of herbs in the management of asthma. *Phcog Rev*. 2009;3:p.247-58

Prazuck T, Tall F, Nacro B, Rochereau A, Traore A, Sanou T, Malkin J E, Apaire-Marchais V, Masson D, Dublanchet et al. HIV Infection and Severe Malnutrition: A Clinical and Epidemiological Study in Burkina Faso. *AIDS*. 1993;Jan:7(1):p.103-8.

Price M L. *The Moringa Tree*. ECHO Technical Note. Educational Concerns for Hunger Organization. N. Ft. Meyers, FL. 1985.

Quisimbing E. *Medicinal Plants of the Philippines*. Katha Publishing Co Inc. Quezon City. 1978;p.346-349.

Radiation Exposure of the U.S. Population from Consumer Products and Miscellaneous Sources Report No. 95. National Council on Radiation Protection and Measurements. Bethesda MD. 1987.

Rajendhran J, Mani M A, et al. Antibacterial activity of some selected medicinal plants. *Geobios Jodhpur*. 1998;25(4): p.280-282.

Ram J. *Moringa a highly nutritious vegetable tree*. Tropical Rural and Island/Atoll Development Experimental Station (TRIADES), Technical Bulletin No.2. 1994.

Ramachandran C, Peter K V, Gopalakrishnan P K. 1980, Drumstick (*Moringa oleifera*): A multipurpose Indian Vegetable. *Economic Botany*, 34 (3) p.276-283.

Randhawa G K, Kullar J S, Rajkumar. Bioenhancers from mother nature and their applicability in modern medicine. *Int J App Basic Med Res*. 2011;1:p.5-10.

Rao A V, Devi P U, Kamath R. In vivo radioprotective effect of *Moringa oleifera* leaves. *Indian J Ex Biol*. 2001;39:p.858-863.

Rao K N V, Gopalakrishnan V, Loganathan V, Shanmuganathan S. Antiinflammatory activity of *Moringa oleifera* Lam. *Ancient Science of Life*. 1999;18(3-4):p.195-198.

Rao Kurma S, Mishra S H. (1993) Drumstick polysaccharide as pharmaceutical adjuvant. *Indian J Natural Products* 1993;9(1): p.3-6.

Rao K S, Misra S H. Anti-inflammatory and antihepatotoxic activities of the rats of Moringa pterygosperma. *Geaertn Ind J Pharma Sci.* 1998;60:p.12-16.

Rao P P, Acharya B M, Dennis T J. Pharmacogniostic study on stembark of *Moringa oleifera* Lam. (Sigru). *B.M.E.B.R.* 1996;17(3-4): p.141-151.

Rathi B, Patil P A, Baheti A M. Evaluation of aqueous extract of pulp and seeds of *Moringa oleifera* for wound healing in albino rats. J Natural Remedies 2004;4:p.145-9.

Ray K, Hazrai R, Guha D. Central inhibitory effect of *Moringa oleifera* root extract: possible role of neurotransmitters. Indian J Exp Biol. 2003; Nov;41 (11):p.1279-84.

Raz I, Rosengarten Y, Carasso R. Correlational study between conventional medical diagnosis and the diagnosis by reflexology (non conventional). Harefuah. 2003; Sep; 142 (8-9): p600-605, 646.

Reddy N S, Bhatt G. Contents of minerals in green leafy vegetables cultivated in soil fortified with different chemical fertilizers. Plant Foods for Human Nutrition. 2001;56:p.1-6.

Ruckmani K, Kavimani S, et al. Effect of Moringa oleifera Lam. on paracetamol-induced hepatotoxicity. Indian Journal of Pharmaceutical Sciences. 1998;60(1):p.33-35.

Ruckmani K, Davimani S, Jayakar B, Anandan R. Anti-ulcer activity of the alkali preparation of the root and fresh leaf juice of Moringa oleifera Lam. Ancient Science of Life. 1998;17(3): p.220-223.

Ruggiero C, Lattanzio F, Lauretani F, et al. Omega-3 polyunsaturated fatty acids and immune-mediated dieases: inflammatory bowel disease and rheumatoid arthritis. Curr Pharm Des. 2009;15(36):p.4135-4138.

Saadabi A M, Abu Zaid I E. An in vitro antimicrobial activity of Moringa oleifera L. seed extracts against different groups of microorgamisms. Aust J of Basic & App Sciences. 2011;5(5):p.129-134.

Sachan A, Meena A K, Kaur R, Pal B, Singh B. Moringa oleifera: A Review. J Pharm Res. 2010;3:p.840-842.

Sairam T V. Home Remedies: A Handbook of Herbal Cures for Common Ailments. Penguin. New Delhi, India. 1999.

Sales C, Oliviero F, Spinella P. The Mediterranean diet model in inflammatory rheumatic diseases. Reumatismo. 2009;61(1):p.10-14.

Sampson W. Studying herbal remedies. NEJM. 2005;353(4):p.337-339.

Sánchez-Machado D I, Núñez-Gastélum J A, C, Reyes-Moreno C, Ramiréz-Wong B, López-Cervantes J. Nutritional quality of edible parts of Moringa oleifera. Food Analytic Methods. 2010;3(3)p.175-180.

Sapolsky R. Biology and Human Behavior: The Neurological Origins of Individuality. (2nd ed.). The Teaching Company. 2005.

Seddon J M, Ajani U A, Sperduto R D, et al.Dietary carotenoids, vitamins A, C, and E, and advanced age-related macular degeneration. Eye Disease Case-Control Study Group. JAMA. 1994; 272(18):p.1413-20

Selgrade M K, Coopr G S, Germolec D R, Heindel J J. Linking Environmental agents to autoimmune disease. Environ Health Perspect. 1999; 107: pS5811-S811.

Selye, Hans. Stress without Distress. Philadelphia. Lippincott. 1974.

Sen Gupta K P, Ganguli N C, Bhattacharjee B. (1956) Bacteriological and pharmacological studies of a vibriocidal drug derived from an indigenous source. The Antiseptic. 1956;53(4): p.287-292.

Sena L P, Vanderjagt D J, Rivera C, Tsin A T, Muhamadu I, Mahamadou O, Millson M, Pastuszyn A, Glew R H. (1998) Analysis of nutritional components of eight famine foods of the Republic of Niger. Plant Foods and Human Nutrition 1998;52:p.17-30.

Serra V, Grune T, Sitte N, Saretzki G, von Zglinicki T. Telomere length as a marker of oxidative stress in primary human fibroblast cultures. Annals of the New York Academy of Sciences. 2000;908:p.327-330.

Shaw B P, Jana P. Clinical assessment of Sigru (*Moringa oelifera* Lam) on Mutrakrichra (lower urinary tract infection) *NAGARJUN*. 1982;p.231-235.

Shukla S, Mathur R, Prakash A O. Biochemical and physiological alterations in female reproductive organs of cyclic rats treated with aqueous extract of *Moringa oleifera* Lam. *Acta Europaea Fertilitatis*. 1988;19: p.225-232.

Shukla S, Mathur R, Prakash A O, et al. (1988) Anti-implantation efficacy of *Moringa oleifera* Lam. and *Moringa concanensis* Nimmo in rats. *International Journal Of Crude Drug Research*. 1988;26(1): p.29-32.

Shukla S, Mathur R, Prakash A O. Antifertility profile of the aqueous extract of *Moringa oleifera* roots. *Journal of Ethnopharmacology*. 1988;22: p.51-62.

Shukla S, Mathur R, Prakash A O. Histoarchitecture of the genital tract of ovariectomized rats treated with an aqueous extract of *Moringa oleifera* roots. *Journal of Ethnopharmacology*. 1989;25: p.249-261.

Shukla S, Mathur R, et al. Biochemical alterations in the female genital tract of ovariectomized rats treated with aqueous extract of *Moringa oleifera* Lam. *Pakistan Journal of Scientific and Industrial Research*. 1989;32(4): p.273-277.

Siddhuraju P, Becker K. Antioxidant properties of various solvent extracts of total phenolic constituents from three different agroclimatic origins of drumstick tree (*Moringa oleifera* Lam.) leaves. *Journal of Agricultural and Food Chemistry*. 2003;51:p. 2144-2155.

Silverstone L M. *Significance of Infrared Energy to Human Health*. <http:www.21stcip.com/pages/silverstone.html.

Simon J A, Fong J, Bernert J T Jr, et al. Serum fatty acids and the risk of stroke. *Stroke*. 1995;26:p.778–782.

Simone C. *Cancer & Nutrition*. Garden City Park, New York. Avery Publishing Group. 1992.

Simopoulis A P. The importance of the ratio of omega-6/omega-3 essential fatty acids. *Biomedicine and Pharmacotherapy*. 2002;56:p.365-379.

Singh K K, Kumar K. Ethnotherapeutics of some medicinal plants used as antipyretic agents among the tribals of India. *Journal of Economic and Taxonomic Botany*. 1999;23(1): p.135-141.

Singha P, Begum J, et al. *Antibacterial activity of some higher plants of Chittagong University Campus*. Chittagong University Studies Part II Science. 1993; 17(1): p.97-101.

Smith L, Purdy-Lloyd K, Phelps K. Biological terrain assessment results of 14 subjects before and after testing with a supplement containing silicon bonded to reduced hydrogen atoms. *J Amer Coll Nutr*. Vol 17 No. 5. 1998; p522.

Soni P L. Some commercially important Indian gum exudates. *Indian Forester*. 1995;121(8): p.754-759

Soyka F. *The Ion Effect*. Bantam Premium. United States. 1991.

Sozou P D, Kirkwood T B. A stochastic model of cell replicative senescence based on telomere shortening,oxidative stress, and somatic mutations in nuclear and mitochondrial DNA. *J Theoretical Biology*.2001;213:p.573-576.

Spiliotis V, Lalas S, et al. Comparison of antimicrobial activity of seeds of different *Moringa oleifera* varieties. *Pharmaceutical and Pharmacological Letters*. 1998;8(1): 39-40.

Stavrovskaia I G, Sirota T V, Saakian I R, Kondrashova M N. Optimization of energy-dependent processes in mitochondria from rat liver and brain after inhalation of negative air ions. *Biofizika*. 1998 Sep-Oct. 43(5):p766-771.

Stechmiller J K et al. Argenine supplementation and wound healing. *Nutrition in Clinical Practice*.2005;20(13):p.52-61.

Stoff J. *An Examination of immune Response Modulation in Humans by Antigen Infused Dialyzable Bovine Colostrum/Whey Extract Using A Double Blind Study*. Tucson. Immune Consultants. 2001.

Stoff J. *A Study of the Effects of Oral Dietary Supplementation of Antigen Infused Colostrum/Whey Extract Upon Natural Killer Cell Activity in a Healthy Human Population*. Scottsdale. Quantum Research Inc. 2001.

Stoff J. *The Ultimate Nutrient*. Tucson. Insight Consulting Services. 2000.

Suarez M, Entenza J M, Doerries C, Meyer E, Bourquin L, Sutherland J, et al. Expression of a plant-derived peptide harboring water-cleaning and antimicrobial activities. Biotechnol Bioeng. 2003;81:p.13-20.

Suarez M, Haenni M, Canarelli S, Fisch F, Chodanowski P, Servis C, et al. Structure-function characterization and optimization of a plant-derived antibacterial peptide. Antimicrob Agents Chemother. 2005;49:p.3847-57.

Subadra S, Monica J, et al. Retention and storage stability of beta-carotene in dehydrated drumstick leaves (Moringa oleifera). International Journal of Food Sciences and Nutrition. 1997;48(6): p.373-379.

Sutar N G, Patil V V, Deshmukh T A, Jawle N M, Patil V R, Bhangale S C. Evaluation of anti-pyretic potential of seeds of Moringa oleifera Lam. Int J Green Pharm. 2009;3:p.148-50.

Sutar N G, Bonde C G, Patil V V, Narkhede S B, Patil A P, Kakade R T. Analgesic activity of seeds of Moringa oleifera Lam. IJGP. 2008;2(2):p.108-110.

Swartz M N. "Hospital acquired infections: diseases with increasingly limited therapies". Proc Natl Acad Sci USA. 1994; 91(7): p.2420-27.

Tabassum N, Ahmad F. Role of natural herbs in the treatment of hypertension. 2011;5:p.30-40.

Tahiliani P, Kar A. Role of Moringa oleifera leaf extract in the regulation of thyroid hormone status in adult male and female rats. Pharmacol Res. 2000; Mar; 41 (3):p.319-23

Talalay P, Talalay P. (2001) The importance of using scientific principles in the development of medicinal agents from plants. Academic Medicine. 2001;76(3): p.238-247.

Tarafder C R. Ethnogynecology in relation to plants: 2. Plants used for abortion. Journal of Economic and Taxonomic Botany 1983;4(2): p.507-516.

Teitlebaum Jacob. From Fatigued to Fantastic! Garden City Park, New York. Avery Publishing Group. 1996.

Terra, G J A. Tropical vegetables, vegetable growing in the tropics and subtropics especially of indigenous vegetables. Communications No. 54e of the Department of Agricultural Research; Publication of the Royal Tropical Institute, Amsterdam, The Netherlands. 1966.

135

The Inside Story: A Guide to Indoor Air Quality. United States Environmental Protection Agency and the United States Consumer Product safety Commission Office of Radiation and Indoor Air (6604J). EPA Document #402-K-93-007. April 1995.

Toyokawa H, Matsui Y, Uhara J, et al. Promotive effects of Far-Infrared Ray on Full-Thickness Skin Wound Healing in Rats. *Experimental Biology and Medicine.* 2003; 228: p724-729.

Tsaknis J, Lalas S, Gergis V, Douroglou V, Spiliotis V. Characterization of *Moringa oleifera* variety Mbololo seed oil of Kenya. *Journal of Agricultural and Food Chemistry.* 1999;47: p.4495-4499.

Tsaknis J, Spiliotis, V. Quality changes of *Moringa oleifera*, variety Mbololo of Kenya, seed oil during frying. *Grasas y Aceites.* 1999;50(1): p.37-48.

Twomey JJ, Good RA, eds. *The Immunopathology of Lymphoreticular Neoplasms.* New York. Plenum Publishing. 1978; p203

Udupa S L, Udupa, A L. A comparative study on the effect of some indigenous drugs on normal and steroid-depressed healing. *Fitoterapia* 1998;69(6): p.507-510.

Udupa S L, Udupa A L et al. Studies on the anti-inflammatory and wound healing properties of *Moringa oleifera* and *Aegle marmelos. Fitoterapia.* 1994;65(2): p.119-123.

U.S. Environmental Protection Agency. *Health Assessment Document for Nickel. 83/012F.* National Center for Environmental Assessment, Office of Research and Development. Washington, DC. 1986.

Verdcourt B. A synopsis of the Moringaceae. *Kew Bulletin.* 1985;40: p.1-23.

Villasenor I M. Bioactive metabolites from *Moringa oleifera.* Lam. *KIMIKA.* 1994;10: p.47-52.

Villasenor I M, Lim-Sylianco C Y, Dayrit F.(1989) Mutagens from roasted seeds of *Moringa oleifera. Mutation Research.* 1989;224: 209-212.

Villasenor I M, Finch P, Lim-Sylianco C Y, Dayrit F. Structure of a mutagen from roasted seeds of *Moringa oleifera. Carcinogenesis.* 1989; 10: p.1085-1087.

Vojdani A, Ghoneum M, Brautbar N. Immune alteration associated with exposure to toxic chemicals. *Toxicol Ind Health*. 1992; 8:p239-253.

Warhurst A M, Raggett S L, McConnachie G L, Pollard S J T, Chipofya V, Codd G A. Adsorption of the cyanobacterial hepatotoxin Microcystin-LR by a low-cost activated carbon from the seed husks of the pan-tropical tree, *Moringa oleifera*. *The Science of the Total Environment*. 1997;207: p.207-211.

Whiteside T et al. Human Natural Killer Cells in health and disease. *Clinical Immunotherapy*. 1994; 1(1)56-66.

Whiteside T, Herberman R. The role of natural killer cells in human disease. *Clin Immunology Immunopathology*. 1989; 53: p1-23.

Williams F, Robertson R, Roworth M. Detailed Profile of 25 major organic and inorganic substances. *Scottish Centre for Infection and Environmental Health*. Glasgow. 1999; 1st ed.

William F, S Lakshminarayanan, et al. Effect of some Indian vegetables on the glucose and insulin response in diabetic subjects. *International Journal of Food Sciences and Nutrition*. 1993; 44(3): p.191-196.

Wright J E, Ed. Charged for Recovery: Negative ions have a positive effect on muscle recuperation. *Muscle & Fitness*. Oct. 1993. Vol 54 no 10.

Yanaka A, Zhang S, Yamamoto M, Fahey J W. Daily intake of sulforaphane-rich broccoli sprouts improves gastritis in *H.pylori*-infected human subjects. *Cancer Epidemiology Biomarkers and Prevention*. 2005; 14(11, Suppl): p.2754s.

Yoo B H, Park C M, Oh T J, Han S H, Kang H H, Chang I S. Investigation of jewelry powders radiating far-infrared rays and the biological effects on human skin. *J Cosmet Sci*. 2002. May-June; 53(3): p175-184.

Yongbai K A. Studies on the potential use of medicinal plants and macrofungi (lower plants) in water and waste water purification. 2005; www.biotech.kth.se/iobb/news/kenneth04.doc.

Yashodhara B M, Umakanth S, Pappachan J M, Bhat S K, Kamath R, Choo B H. Omega-3 fatty acids: a comprehensive review of their role in health and disease. *Postgrad Med J*. 2009;86(1000):p.84-90.

Zainal Z, Longman AJ, Hurst S, et al. Relative efficacies of omega-3 polyunsaturated fatty acids in reducing expression of key proteins in a model system for studying osteoarthritis. *Osteoarthritis Cartilage*. 2009;17(7):p.896-905.

ABOUT THE AUTHOR

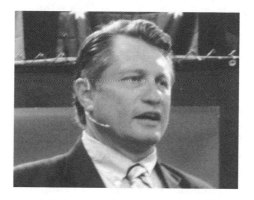

Dr. Howard W. Fisher,

Dr. Howard Fisher is a natural physician specializing in Anti-Aging medicine who is on a mission to educate and enlighten the world about the toxic factors that exist in our environment and their direct relationship to our health. His current seminar that he delivers to both Medical Anti-Aging Conferences and medical schools world-wide, makes both professionals and the public aware of the omnipresent threats present in our immediate environment and gives insightful plans of remediation. Dr. Howard W. Fisher is a member of the Scientific Review Committee of the Dubai Congress on Anti-Aging & Aesthetic Medicine. He has special interests in anti-aging, immunology, electromagnetic radiation and nutrition, and this researching author acts as a consultant and educator for several multi-national nutritional companies and has advised several governments on electromagnetic radiation effects. Dr. Fisher lectures internationally on anti-aging, nutrition, wellness, and immunology. He has written many articles for trade publications and is a featured guest on many radio and television broadcasts. In addition to authoring thirteen health oriented books, his research has also been published in peer-reviewed journals. His books and lectures have been translated into seven languages and are sold in North America, Europe and Asia.

Being widely recognized for his ability to easily assimilate what many view as daunting scientific and clinical information, Dr. Fisher transforms essential knowledge that would otherwise remain inaccessible to the public into readily available life-altering information. The foundation of his philosophy rests upon understanding and exposing the true nutritional and environmental deficiencies that exist in our everyday lives, and scouring the planet for the most efficient solutions to not only solving these threatening health issues, but improving the well-being and overall quality of life for everyone. His common sense approach to explaining the impact of our environmental factors to the health of the world makes it easy for his audience to make informed choices towards bettering their lives.

In addition to his research, writing and lecturing, Dr. Fisher is still an avid athlete who runs, plays hockey, and can be found on the golf course most mornings. A dynamic and colorful personality, Dr. Fisher resides in Toronto, Ontario with his wife and two children when not lecturing abroad.

OTHER BOOKS BY
DR. HOWARD W. FISHER

Wisdom of the Woods: Herbal Remedies

Extreme Toxic Times: How to Escape On Your Own
Two Feet

Reishi Rescue: R & R for Your Immune System

Before You Breathe Deeply: The Immunological
Significance of Breathing Purified Air

Nature's Silver Bullet: Killing the Fear Factor
Reishi Response: Answering Today's Health Challenges

Approaching Wellness: Simple Steps to Restore Your
Immune System

Enzymes and Your Health: Optimizing Your
Physiological Functions

The Invisible Threat : The Risks Associated With EMFs

The Invisible Threat II: A Solution to the EMF
Radiation Crisis.

Molecular Resonance Effect Technology: The
Dynamic Effects on Human Physiology

Optimal Hydration the Key to Health and Anti-Aging

To find out more about Dr. Fisher's upcoming lectures
or books go to www.fisherclinic.com

NOTES

NOTES

NOTES